D1033165

THE

HARVARD MEDICAL

SCHOOL GUIDE TO

Healthy Eating
During Pregnancy

YOLO COUNTY LIBRARY
226 BUCKEYE STREET
WOODLAND, CA 95695

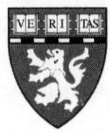

THE

HARVARD MEDICAL

SCHOOL GUIDE TO

Healthy Eating

During Pregnancy

W. Allan Walker, M.D.

with Courtney Humphries

McGraw·Hill

New York   Chicago   San Francisco   Lisbon   London   Madrid   Mexico City
Milan   New Delhi   San Juan   Seoul   Singapore   Sydney   Toronto

The McGraw·Hill Companies

Library of Congress Cataloging-in-Publication Data

Walker, W. Allan.
   The Harvard Medical School guide to healthy eating during pregnancy / W. Allan
   Walker with Courtney Humphries.
        p.   cm.
   Includes bibliographical references and index.
   ISBN 0-07-144332-0
        1. Pregnancy—Nutritional aspects—Popular works.   2. Pregnant women—
   health and hygiene—Popular works.   I. Humphries, Courtney.   II. Title.
   III. Title: Guide to healthy eating during pregnancy.

   RG559.W35   2006
   618.2'42—dc22   2005030234

Copyright © 2006 by The President and Fellows of Harvard College. All rights reserved.
Printed in the United States of America. Except as permitted under the United States
Copyright Act of 1976, no part of this publication may be reproduced or distributed in any
form or by any means, or stored in a database or retrieval system, without the prior written
permission of the publisher.

1 2 3 4 5 6 7 8 9 0   DOC/DOC   0 9 8 7 6 5

ISBN 0-07-144332-0

Illustrations on pages 22–23 by Scott Leighton, on pages 66–67 by Christopher Bing, on
page 123 by Matthew Holt, and on page 175 by Patrick Scullin.

McGraw-Hill books are available at special quantity discounts to use as premiums and
sales promotions, or for use in corporate training programs. For more information, please
write to the Director of Special Sales, Professional Publishing, McGraw-Hill, Two Penn
Plaza, New York, NY 10121-2298. Or contact your local bookstore.

The information contained in this book is intended to provide helpful and informative
material on the subject addressed. It is not intended to serve as a replacement for
professional medical advice. Any use of the information in this book is at the reader's
discretion. The author, publisher, and the President and Fellows of Harvard College
specifically disclaim any and all liability arising directly or indirectly from the use or
application of any information contained in this book. A health-care professional should
be consulted regarding your specific situation.

This book is printed on acid-free paper.

I dedicate this book to my daughter, Dr. Kim Walker;
my daughter-in-law, Heather McDonald Walker;
and my nieces, Dr. Beth Eames Littlejohn and Pam Henley—
all of whom have recently delivered healthy, full-term newborns.

Contents

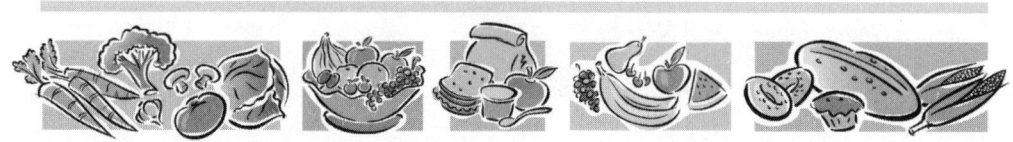

Preface

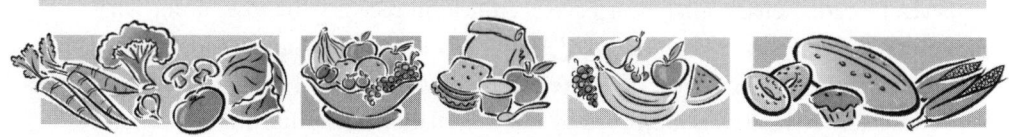

In 2005, McGraw-Hill published our book *Eat, Play, and Be Healthy*, which summarized what is known, scientifically, about what constitutes a healthy diet for infants and young children. A *child's* diet can have important and lasting health effects—for good and bad.

It may seem hard to believe, but recent research reveals that what a *mother* eats during pregnancy can affect whether her child will develop diseases such as heart disease and diabetes—forty to fifty years later, when that child is an adult.

Women who have poor nutrition or weight problems during pregnancy are more likely to give birth to babies who are not at their optimal weight at birth, and birth weight has been shown to play an important role in health into adulthood. Research has shown that you can improve your child's health if you do the following:

- Reach a healthy weight before becoming pregnant
- Follow a balanced diet and boost key nutrients before conception
- Avoid gaining too little or too much weight while you're pregnant
- Nourish yourself with a balanced diet with the right nutrients
- Stay active during your pregnancy

This book tells you what you need to know about healthy eating while you are pregnant so that you can give your child the best start on a healthy life. You will learn about the science of pregnancy while also getting sound, practical advice about nutrition and health before, during, and after your pregnancy.

The recent widespread interest in nutrition early in life—from conception to birth and into infancy and early childhood—stems in part from exciting observations made by Dr. David Barker and his associates from Birmingham, England. Several international conferences have been held in recent years to examine what we know about this subject and to identify the additional research that is needed in this important new area. The latest conference, held in November 2005 in Bethesda, Maryland, was sponsored by the U.S. National Institute of Child Health and Human Development (NICHD) at the National Institutes of Health. Experts in the field of obstetrics, public health, perinatology, and nutrition met to review the current evidence for nutrition during pregnancy. Attending that conference helped give us the impetus to write this book.

Much additional research is under way. One of the most exciting projects is being conducted here at Harvard Medical School. Researchers are analyzing data obtained from children born to participants in the famous Nurses' Health Study, and they should have important findings to report in the foreseeable future. NICHD is establishing a large-scale database of newborn infants from various ethnic and racial backgrounds to identify the factors that can predict adult disease. Through studies such as these, we hope to learn about nutrition's role in health from conception to adolescence.

The information in this book is consistent with the nutritional policy statements issued by the Committee of Nutrition of the American Academy of Pediatrics, the most influential body for advising pediatricians on appropriate nutritional care for children.

My own interest in children's nutrition and the need for establishing healthy eating habits early in life stems back to my undergraduate, premedical days at a small midwestern liberal arts college, DePauw University. As a participant in a service project in my senior year, I worked with welfare agencies in Indianapolis to help prevent malnutrition and subsequent infection among inner-city children. This happened in the days before the U.S. government established the Special Supplemental Nutrition Program for Women, Infants, and Children (known as WIC) and the School Lunch Nutrition Program to offer federal support to nutritionally needy kids.

My interest in infant nutrition continued when as a medical student at Washington University School of Medicine in St. Louis, Missouri, I delivered milk to inner-city kids in Chicago. As a resident and chief resident in pediatrics at the University of Minnesota teaching hospital in Minneapolis, Minnesota, I became interested in how the digestive system develops in newborns and the role that nutrition plays in keeping them healthy. After my residency, I trained at Massachusetts General Hospital (MGH) in gastroenterology and nutrition and established the first Pediatric Gastroenterology and Nutrition Division at that hospital. In the early 1980s, I was asked to merge the two pediatric gastroenterology and nutrition programs at Harvard (one based at Children's Hospital Boston and the other at Massachusetts General Hospital for Children) into a combined training program for pediatricians. During the past twenty years, I've helped train many, if not most, of the pediatric nutritionists in academic centers throughout North America and Europe. As leader of one of seven National Institutes of Health–funded Clinical Nutrition Research Centers, I study how nutrition influences the development of intestinal allergies and intestinal immune defenses against infections.

My ultimate goal is to help improve children's health by encouraging better nutrition through research and education. But this goal has increasingly brought me to the field of maternal health, because the two are inextricably linked. You can give your child a boost toward a healthy life during your pregnancy. Our goal in writing this book is to let you know how you can do that. I hope you think we have succeeded.

Acknowledgments

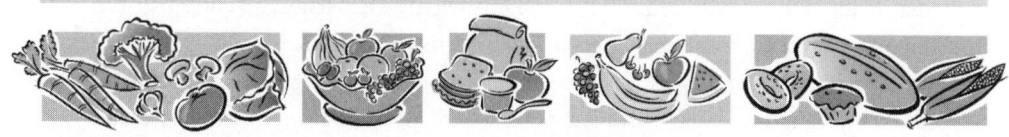

Many people and institutions made this book possible. I am grateful to Harvard Medical School and Massachusetts General Hospital for their institutional support. Harvard Medical School recognized the importance of nutrition in health by establishing a schoolwide Division of Nutrition (DON) in 1996, and I was asked to be its first director. The intent of establishing this division was to give more recognition to nutrition in medicine and to coordinate the large but diffuse resources in nutrition at the medical school and its major teaching hospitals. At the request of numerous graduating classes of the medical school, the DON has aimed to teach practical information about nutrition to Harvard medical students to help create physicians who are more knowledgeable regarding the importance of nutrition in medical practice. Harvard Medical School and Massachusetts General Hospital, where I practice pediatrics, recognized the importance of this field by creating an endowed chair, the Conrad Taff Professorship of Nutrition and Pediatrics, which I am honored to hold.

Courtney Humphries drafted the book in clear and engaging prose and demonstrated a remarkable facility for explaining complicated concepts in a simple way. She eliminated my "medicalese" and straightened out my syntax.

Many individuals have reviewed portions of this book—experts, potential readers (women of childbearing age), and many who were both. Drs. Emily Oken and

Matt Gillman, experts on intrauterine programming at Harvard Medical School and Harvard School of Public Health, reviewed the most complex chapter (Chapter 3) for accuracy. Dr. Carine Lenders, at Children's Hospital Boston and Boston City Hospital, and Dr. Alison Hoppin, at Massachusetts General Hospital for Children—experts for optimal weight for life programs—provided a review of the factual content of this book. Dr. Chris Duggan also provided valuable advice.

Dr. Kim Walker, a child psychologist and my daughter; Dr. Beth Littlejohn, a pediatric endocrinologist and my niece; Dr. Helen Delichatsios, an internist; Dr. Annemarie Broderick, a pediatric gastroenterologist; Sharon Collier, dietary director of the Nutrition Support Service at Children's Hospital; Heather McDonald Walker, my daughter-in-law; and Kirsten Steward Beckwith, a mother of two and a self-taught expert on perinatal nutrition, all reviewed early chapters for readability and clarity. Each of them is a recent mother.

Julie Redfern, a well-known nutritionist in obstetrics at the Brigham and Women's Hospital, reviewed and provided practical dietary suggestions for the recipes in Chapter 9. This is particularly true for suggested healthy snacks and easily prepared but balanced meals. I also wish to thank Lisa F. O'Gorman, a certified executive chef, for the practical recipes provided to parents wishing to make healthy meals during their pregnancy and healthy school lunches for their children. Chris Just, a registered nurse and certified nurse midwife, and Elizabeth Noble, an author and physical therapist, provided practical information about exercises during pregnancy.

Dr. Anthony Komaroff, editor-in-chief; Nancy Ferrari, managing editor; and Christine Junge, editor, of the Harvard Health Publications Division of Harvard Medical School provided important support and encouragement in the development of this book. Judith McCarthy, publisher at McGraw-Hill, helped enormously in editing and organizing this book.

As always, I am grateful to my wife, Dr. Ann Sattler, who is also a pediatrician and mother, for her encouragement and support of my many activities in pediatric nutrition. I also thank my children—Kim, Mike, Andy, and Meredith—and my grandchildren—Douglas, Lena, and Giselle—for keeping me honest in my suggestions for practical approaches to developing healthy eating habits during childhood.

Introduction

Good Nutrition Begins Before Birth

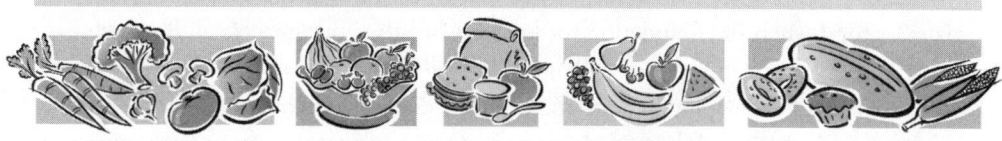

When does good nutrition become important in our lives? For some people, nutrition may not enter their concerns until they are well into adulthood, when they begin worrying that the foods they eat may increase their risk of developing diabetes or heart disease. Others worry about nutrition only when it causes them to gain weight as their metabolism slows with age. For parents, the first time they may become aware of their children's nutrition is when their babies first start eating solid foods. Then there are decisions to make. Which foods are best? Should my baby or small child eat sweets? Is my picky child eating enough of the right kinds of foods to grow? The decisions become more complicated as babies become toddlers and start making demands and refusals for food, and parents must balance their children's wishes with what's good for their health. And as children get older and go to school, they are more influenced by peers, the media, and the food available at school, and suddenly nutrition can become a major issue in parents' minds.

In fact, in this book I'm going to argue that good nutrition starts in the womb. Your role as a prospective parent begins with the choices you make while you're pregnant. We used to think that babies grow and develop inside their mothers about the same way regardless of the mothers' health and nutrition. A fetus, it was thought, would simply feed upon the reserves of energy and nutrients stored in its mother's body and get everything it needed from her internal supplies. Now we know that that picture is not entirely true. How well a mother eats and how she cares for herself make a big difference in the quality of nutrition her baby receives.

If you are reading this book, it's likely that you are either planning a pregnancy or are already pregnant and wondering how to eat well for your baby's health. Congratulations on taking the time to educate yourself about nutrition now, at the beginning of your child's life. Your effort will help to better your own health and the long-term health of your future baby.

A growing body of research is showing that the time a baby spends in the womb is the period when the foundation for her later health is put into place. Research has now shown that the events that happen in fetal life can in part determine a person's chances of developing diseases such as heart disease, high blood pressure, diabetes, and obesity in adulthood. As a mother-to-be, your first step in improving your child's nutrition is to take care of your own health and nutrition before and during pregnancy. By doing so, you will be helping to ensure your child's health at birth and into adulthood.

What's in This Book

This book will help educate you about good nutrition before, during, and after pregnancy. More than just a list of foods to eat or not eat, this book will help you understand the following:

- How to be nutritionally ready for pregnancy
- What happens to your body and your baby's body throughout your pregnancy
- How the behaviors you adopt affect your baby's development
- Why certain foods and dietary habits are healthier than others
- Which nutritional "building blocks" your baby needs from your diet
- How to incorporate healthy weight gain and exercise into your pregnancy
- How to recover from pregnancy, follow good nutrition while nursing, and gradually return to what you weighed before pregnancy

This book is about *your* nutrition, but it's also about *your baby's* nutrition while he is growing inside you. Your baby's nutrition depends not only on the foods you eat but also on how well your body can deliver those nutrients. "Fetal nutrition" relies on the overall health of the mother and her health habits. So I will talk about nutrition broadly, including some of your behaviors and physical activities as well as the foods you eat.

Here is a more detailed look at the contents of this book, chapter by chapter:

If you're not yet pregnant but are planning a pregnancy, you have the opportunity to improve your health now and help prevent pregnancy complications or health problems in your baby. Chapter 1 discusses how you can nutritionally prepare for pregnancy, make sure your weight and nutrition aren't causing infertility problems, eliminate habits that may harm your baby, and make sure your weight is at the healthiest level possible for pregnancy.

Chapter 2 is a brief look at how pregnancy works, what changes occur in your body, and how your baby's growth progresses. Your body will accomplish some amazing things in just nine months, and you are undoubtedly curious about what's happening. This chapter will help satisfy your curiosity.

In Chapter 3, I will share with you some important new research showing that good health begins in the womb and that problems with nutrition during development can have impacts on certain diseases in adulthood. This chapter is heavier on science than the others, but I think it will help readers who are interested in what is known about health and disease understand how research is shaping our view on pregnancy.

Chapter 4 will help you change your diet for the better. I will help you understand how to follow a balanced diet, choose the healthiest foods and avoid unhealthy ones, and pay attention to the nutrients that are particularly needed during pregnancy.

After explaining how to make positive changes in your nutrition, in Chapter 5 I'll review all the habits and substances that may be harmful to your fetus during pregnancy. I'll help you distinguish the habits that should be avoided entirely, such as alcohol and drug use, from those that require caution, such as eating fish that may be contaminated with mercury.

Chapter 6 will discuss dietary supplements, which include any "extras" people add to their diets, such as multivitamins, herbal remedies, and nutritional supplements. I'll help you sort fact from hype and determine which products are useful and which may be dangerous.

Weight gain and weight control are confusing issues in pregnancy, and many women don't get the proper advice they need. Chapter 7 will explain why paying attention to weight gain is important for your health and your baby's, and how you can make sure you're gaining the right amount of weight.

Chapter 8 explains how a pregnant woman can continue to exercise and stay active throughout pregnancy without harming her baby. I'll give you specific stretches and movements that will help target important muscles and problem areas for pregnant women.

Chapter 9 is filled with delicious recipes and eating tips to help you take some of the basic information you've learned and apply it to specific foods in your diet.

After you deliver your baby, you'll undoubtedly be caught up in the joys and concerns of parenting. But there are still some important steps to take for your own health as you recover. In Chapter 10 I'll give you guidance on losing your pregnancy weight and getting your body back in shape. I'll discuss the decision to breast-feed or formula-feed your baby, and I'll help breast-feeding moms follow a nutritious and safe diet while they nurse.

What Do We Really Know?

My goal is to write a book about nutrition during pregnancy that is both useful for pregnant women and built upon strong scientific evidence. It's not as easy as it sounds. People are often confused about nutrition, and pregnancy seems to garner some of the most creative and suspect ideas about what to eat and what not to eat. In talking with my female colleagues and friends, I've heard countless pieces of advice that are passed from person to person about how to be healthy during pregnancy. I've also attended conferences and lectures about maternal nutrition during pregnancy, where I've heard leading experts talk about how we still have much to learn about how pregnancy works and how a mother's nutrition affects her baby.

There's a disconnect here. Mothers want a simple list of what to eat and what not to eat. But scientists still have not answered many basic questions, much less come up with those dietary details that people want to hear. The result is that many books and websites about pregnancy rely on less-than-sound information that is told to women as if it were fact. In this book I hope to be sensitive to your needs for practical advice. But I will also be honest about where the advice comes from, how sound it is, and what is still unknown. Here is a brief overview of the kinds of evidence that shape our ideas about nutrition during pregnancy:

• *Scientific evidence.* When we talk about "evidence-based medicine," we mean that medical decisions are made as much as possible based on information that has been scientifically tested and proved. But while new drugs and treatments can be tested rigorously before they get out to the public, none of us can avoid eating until all the evidence comes in on what a healthy diet is. Medical and health organizations often compile recommendations for diet that are based on the best available evidence, and I have relied on these recommendations wherever possible.

- *Clinical experience.* Scientific studies are expensive to conduct, can take years to complete, and often cannot fully answer a particular question until several studies are conducted. Working physicians, nurses, and nutritionists can't always wait for definitive scientific proof before choosing a course of action for their patients. Instead they rely on past experience and on the advice and experience of their mentors and colleagues—often called empirical evidence. Many recommendations for nutrition are based on experience, on what seems to work, and on what fits with our common sense. There's nothing wrong with following common sense in choosing what to eat, but it's important to keep in mind that the advice we give may change if more rigorous scientific studies prove our assumptions wrong.

- *Animal studies.* Pregnancy is such a delicate and vulnerable time that there are only limited ways to study pregnancy in a human woman ethically and safely. Much of what we know about how pregnancy works comes from studying animals. We know that there are significant differences between the way humans work and the way other animals work, so animal studies cannot be taken at face value. But if an animal study points to a particular way of thinking about pregnancy, it can add strength to a hypothesis or help guide further research in humans.

- *Anecdotes, myths, and urban legend.* The lowest level of recommendation is one based simply on an isolated example or an "urban legend" that has been passed from person to person but hasn't been tested or verified. This is the kind of advice that many people hear and I'd like to avoid.

Pregnancy Is a Great Time to Change for the Better

For many women, pregnancy may be the first time they really begin to examine their health habits and question how their diet affects their body. Knowing that their children are directly affected by the foods they eat suddenly makes good nutrition seem much more important than it used to seem. Most women are even willing to give up foods they like or adopt new habits to ensure the health of their babies. But what happens after pregnancy? Is your health any less important once you are no longer carrying a baby inside of you?

I'd like you to view your pregnancy as a time to make changes for the better—lasting changes that you can take with you into your life as a mother after pregnancy. If you can learn to eat healthier for your baby, why not continue eating healthier for yourself? Not only will long-term changes help you live a longer life free of disease, but it will ultimately benefit your children and your family to have you in the best health possible. Some of the information in this book applies specifically to pregnancy. But the overall approach to a healthy lifestyle can apply anytime in your life. In the last chapter, I'll explain some of the ways you can apply good eating habits to your life after pregnancy and thereby lower your risk of chronic disease and health problems in the future.

Healthy Mothers, Healthy Babies

The purpose of this book is to help women who are pregnant or planning a pregnancy acquire the tools they need to stay healthy and nourish themselves as best they can. But it's also important to realize that many of the factors that can lead to pregnancy complications and poor health in babies are largely outside of women's control. These include genetics, poverty, lack of adequate health care, violence, drug or alcohol addiction, and exposure to environmental toxins and pollutants. In addition to the personal choices we make about our health, social and environmental factors have a great impact on our health and our children's health. In spite of our singular wealth and resources, the United States ranks twenty-eighth in the world in infant mortality, largely because of our disparities in health care along racial and socioeconomic lines. A book like this can, unfortunately, reach only a subset of women, and it can address only the factors under their control. We also need good support services and outreach programs to give resources, education, and access to good nutrition to all women. Every society has an investment in the health of its citizens. Helping women stay healthy benefits their health as well as the health of our next generation of children.

How to Find More Information

This book is intended to provide the latest scientifically based information on nutrition during pregnancy. I have included references to books, articles, and websites where you can find more information on the topics covered here. This book is not meant to substitute for individualized care from your physician and is not a comprehensive guide to your health during pregnancy. If you have medical questions or experience pain or other unusual symptoms during your pregnancy, always alert your doctor first. While your obstetrician can offer some guidance on nutrition, speaking with a registered dietitian (RD) can be invaluable if you are seeking further information or require a special nutrition plan for a medical condition. The RD credential is issued by the Commission on Accreditation for Dietetics Education of the American Dietetic Association (ADA) to applicants who have completed special course work and a supervised practice program and have passed a national examination. Hospitals and clinics often have RDs on staff, some of whom may specialize in prenatal nutrition. You can also find a registered dietitian in your area through the ADA's website at eatright.org.

For more general information on nutrition, the U.S. Department of Health and Human Services and the Department of Agriculture recently issued revised Dietary Guidelines for Americans that include specific suggestions for weight management along with information about diet, reflecting a growing recognition that the two are inextricably linked in a healthy lifestyle. The guidelines also single out the needs of specific populations, including pregnant women. A summary of the key recommendations are available at this website: health.gov/dietaryguidelines/dga2005 /document/html/executivesummary.htm. After your pregnancy, I also recommend Walter C. Willett's book *Eat, Drink, and Be Healthy* for science-based advice on a healthy diet for adults. And my book *Eat, Play, and Be Healthy* applies this knowledge to the special needs of your children, from infancy to age eight. Helpful information is also available from the Harvard School of Public Health's website "Nutrition Source," hsph.harvard.edu/nutritionsource.

THE

HARVARD MEDICAL

SCHOOL GUIDE TO

Healthy Eating

During Pregnancy

1

How to Prepare
for Pregnancy

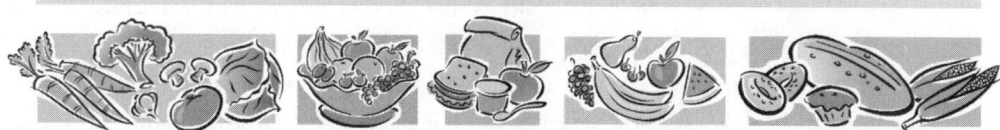

About half of all pregnancies in the United States are unplanned. But increasingly women are able to plan their pregnancies, a trend that has the potential to improve children's health when mothers-to-be take the time to make sure they are entering pregnancy prepared. If you've started to read this book before pregnancy, congratulations; you have the opportunity to take some positive steps to help secure your future baby's health.

Women who are hoping to become pregnant are often concerned with ensuring their fertility, and we'll talk about the role nutrition may play helping you conceive. The goal of planning for pregnancy is not just to help you get pregnant but also to help ensure that you are in the best possible health when you become pregnant. By achieving a good state of health before your pregnancy, you can help avoid some potential complications and also increase the chances that your child will be healthy. Here are a few of the advantages of prepregnancy planning:

- Reaching a healthy weight before pregnancy will make your pregnancy easier and can contribute to the long-term health of your child.
- Supplementing your diet with folic acid now can help prevent birth defects.
- Adopting good health habits now will help you maintain them throughout your pregnancy.
- Getting any medical conditions under control before pregnancy can help prevent complications.

If you are planning a pregnancy, you should start changing habits now rather than waiting until you are pregnant. There are two reasons why it's good to plan ahead. One is simply that changing habits can be a difficult task. The more time you allow yourself to start following a healthier diet, cutting back on harmful habits, and addressing your own health, the easier it will be to have a healthy pregnancy.

The second reason is the unpredictability of pregnancy. Once you start trying to get pregnant, you won't know whether it will happen this week, this month, or this year. You won't know for sure that you are pregnant until you miss a period and have a positive pregnancy test. By that time, you will probably have been pregnant for a couple of weeks or more. While a few weeks is just a small amount of time in a person's life, it is a critical time for your baby's development. Those first weeks are a time when the foundations of a baby's body are put into place; just three days after your first missed period, all of the major organs in your baby's body have begun to form. During this time, your baby's health is sensitive to potential nutri-

Prep Time

How much time should you devote to the preparation period before pregnancy? It will depend on the kinds of changes you need to make. If you need to gain or lose weight (see the section on reaching a healthy weight in this chapter), the more time you can take the better—ideally several months to a year. The same goes for quitting smoking or other addictions. The goal is to establish healthy habits, and that takes time. However, women who are older or otherwise don't have the luxury of taking months or a year to get pregnant can still benefit from spending a month or two focusing on their diet, physical activity level, and eating habits to improve them prior to conceiving.

ent deficiencies or exposures to harmful substances. Because you can't be sure when pregnancy will happen, the best chance to give your baby a healthy start is to make sure you are already providing the proper environment for a fetus before you become pregnant.

Reach a Healthy Weight Before Pregnancy

Weight plays an important role in a healthy pregnancy. Women whose weight is below normal for their height are at a greater risk for premature delivery and having a smaller-than-average baby. Overweight or obese women are at higher risk for having complications during pregnancy, a difficult delivery, and a baby who weighs more than average—and their babies are more likely to have weight problems as adults. As I will explain further in Chapter 3, both of these extremes can lead to stunted growth and development in the womb. Babies who experience growth restriction in the womb have higher risks of developing chronic disease as adults. So an unhealthy weight isn't just a threat to your pregnancy—it is a factor that can influence your child's health into adulthood.

We often have subjective ideas of how much weight is too little or too much. To get a more objective view, find your body mass index (BMI) in the chart provided in Chapter 7. Body mass index is a ratio of weight to height, and it is commonly used in the health field as a more accurate measurement of body size than weight alone. (After all, a man who is six feet four inches tall and weighs two hundred pounds is not overweight, but a man of the same weight who is five feet seven inches tall is overweight.)

The health consequences of being overweight come from being overfat. BMI is not a perfect measurement because it doesn't tell you if the weight you carry is largely muscle or fat. Many bodybuilders fall into the category of overweight even though they may have very little fat, and just because their BMI is high doesn't mean they will be saddled with the same health problems that come with obesity. However, when most of us gain weight it's because we put on excess fat. So BMI is a useful measure of whether your weight is normal or is putting you at risk for health problems.

There are ongoing debates about what BMI is considered normal, overweight, or obese. In general, people agree that a BMI below 26 for women who are planning a pregnancy is a healthy weight, a BMI from 26 to 29 is overweight, and a BMI above 29 is considered obese. Table 1.1 represents the current classifications

Table 1.1   Body Mass Index (BMI) Before Pregnancy

CLASSIFICATION	BMI
Underweight	<19.8
Normal weight	19.8–26.0
Overweight	26.0–29.0
Obese	>29.0

agreed on by the Institute of Medicine based on the best evidence about healthy weight.

The specific cutoffs of these categories make it easier for researchers and health-care workers to classify people and make guidelines, but they can also be misleading. In reality, the health consequences of weight form a spectrum, with potential health risks at either end. People who fall outside the normal range can greatly improve both their chances of conceiving and the health of their pregnancy by reaching a normal weight—or closer to a normal weight—*before they begin trying to conceive.* If you fall outside a normal BMI, talk to your doctor to see whether it is appropriate to set up a plan for gaining or losing weight before pregnancy to get closer to normal.

Underweight Women

It's generally easier for women to gain than to lose, but gaining weight can be a challenge for women who are underweight from severe dieting, eating disorders, or a highly athletic lifestyle. As I'll discuss in the later section on fertility, gaining some weight can also help you conceive in the first place. Your calorie needs grow during pregnancy, and if you have trouble maintaining a healthy weight now, it may be difficult for you to gain the weight you need to throughout pregnancy, especially if you also experience nausea, vomiting, or aversions to certain foods. Don't think about the weight gain itself as the goal; instead, think about gradually increasing the amount of nourishing foods you eat and, if you are an athlete, moderating your exercise levels so you are not expending more energy than you take in. If you have an eating disorder or believe you may have one, seek counseling or treatment in preparation for pregnancy. The undue emphasis our society places on thinness can make it psychologically difficult for many women to gain the weight they need to support a pregnancy, but doing so is critical for your child's health.

Overweight and Obese Women

Weighing too much isn't just a cosmetic problem. Being overweight or obese can lead to serious long-term health problems, including diabetes, heart disease, stroke, gallstones, respiratory problems, and arthritis. In women, obesity can lead to abnormal periods and infertility. Obese women account for one-third of all pregnancies in the United States, and being obese puts women at a higher risk of pregnancy complications such as gestational diabetes, high blood pressure, a difficult labor, or cesarean section. Obese women give birth to larger babies that are more prone to developing diabetes, obesity, and heart disease later in life. A recent population-based study on women in Atlanta also found a higher rate of birth defects among overweight and obese women who gave birth.

If you are overweight or obese, losing about 10 percent of your body weight can improve your chances of conceiving and lower your chances of developing complications in pregnancy. It can reduce the likelihood that your baby will be born with health problems, reduce your child's risk of chronic disease in adulthood, and reduce your own risk of developing chronic disease such as heart disease or diabetes after pregnancy. In fact, reaching a healthier weight before pregnancy is one of the most important steps you can take for your own health—and the health of your future child. The severity of problems increases with BMI, so women who are obese should especially try to get closer to the normal range.

A period of gradual weight loss under a physician's supervision is best. It's far better to lose some weight and then maintain that healthier weight for some time than to lose weight quickly and get pregnant while you are cutting back on calories. Don't compromise your own health by setting goals that are too drastic or unattainable, skipping meals, or trying to follow a fad diet; it's not a good idea to begin a pregnancy with poor nutrition or exhaustion from cutting back on food. Focus on making better food choices, such as the ones suggested later in this chapter and in Chapter 4, rather than eating less food. You are not trying to reach some ideal weight, just improve your health the best you can. If you lose a few pounds over several months but still fall outside of the "healthy weight" range, don't feel frustrated. Even a minor weight loss can have an impact on your baby's health! And small, gradual losses will be easier to maintain over the long term.

Take a Folic Acid Supplement Every Day

The 2005 federal *Dietary Guidelines for Americans* recommend that *all* women of childbearing age take a daily folic acid supplement and eat folic acid–rich foods, because this nutrient is important for preventing birth defects of the brain and spinal cord.

Folic acid, or folate, plays an important role in a fetus's development, particularly the development of the nervous system. The nervous system is one of the first body systems to develop; it begins as a tiny disc of specialized cells in the early embryo. About twenty-six days after conception, this round disc begins to fold over itself and fuse shut, forming a cylinder called the *neural tube*, which is destined to become the brain and spinal cord. If the neural tube fails to close properly, it can lead to birth defects that can be fatal or greatly debilitating—spina bifida, in which the neural tube fails to close at the spine, is the most common nonfatal neural tube defect and can result in nerve damage, lower limb paralysis, and learning disabilities. Folic acid is needed to complete the closure of the neural tube, so women need to have enough folic acid in their bodies available to the fetus. Because the closure of the neural tube happens before many women know they are pregnant, it's very important to begin folic acid supplementation *before* pregnancy.

The federal government launched a program to fortify the food supply with folic acid—particularly breakfast cereals and flour—to raise overall folic acid intake in the American population. Although there is evidence that this program has worked by reducing the incidence of neural tube defects, the amount of folic acid in these foods alone is still not enough to bring you up to adequate levels. It is recommended that women of childbearing years take a folic acid supplement of 400 micrograms daily (as a solitary supplement or part of a multivitamin) while also aiming for an additional 200 micrograms from foods such as those in the following list, for a total of 600 micrograms per day. You can usually achieve 200 micrograms by eating two servings of folate-rich foods per day—see Chapter 4 for folic acid content of selected foods.

High-Folate Foods
Fortified breakfast cereals
Chickpeas (garbanzo beans)
Pinto beans
Lima beans
Asparagus

Spinach
Romaine lettuce
Red kidney beans
Collard greens
Wheat germ
Orange juice

Iron Up

Iron deficiency is the most common nutritional deficiency in the United States and is most common in young children and women of childbearing age, particularly pregnant women. The expansion of your blood volume during pregnancy and the demands of your growing baby put you at higher risk of iron deficiency or anemia, which raises your risk of preterm delivery and having a baby of low birth weight. It can be more difficult to overcome a preexisting iron deficiency during pregnancy because your body's iron needs double during that time.

Your body keeps a small amount of iron in storage. The digestive system helps maintain a balance of iron by absorbing it from foods only when stores become low. Women of childbearing age tend to have lower iron stores because they lose menstrual blood every month. Your iron reserves can become depleted if you don't consume enough iron to refill them. At the most severe level, you can develop anemia, which is characterized by fatigue, irritability, weakness, and shortness of

Start Taking Prenatal Supplements

Although all women should be taking a folic acid supplement before pregnancy, you don't need to take it in isolation. Instead, you can start taking a daily multivitamin or special prenatal vitamin that contains a range of vitamins and minerals needed in pregnancy. These supplements don't substitute for a healthy diet, but they can help prevent any deficiencies. Because you will be taking a daily prenatal supplement during pregnancy, you can start now to get in the habit.

Never take "megadoses" of vitamins beyond the recommended daily intake. Be especially cautious about high levels of vitamin A, which is linked to birth defects.

breath, though some people have no noticeable symptoms of illness. Your doctor should screen you for anemia using a hematocrit or hemoglobin test or, for a more subtle iron deficiency, using a serum ferritin or total iron binding capacity (TIBC) test.

You don't need to take an iron supplement before pregnancy unless recommended by your doctor to overcome a deficiency, but you should aim for two or more servings per day of foods high in iron. Iron that is found in animal products (called *heme iron*) is two to three times more easily absorbed by your body than iron found in plants and iron-fortified foods. For that reason, eating vegetables and other plant foods high in iron is less efficient than eating iron-rich meats. But you can increase how much iron you absorb from plant foods by pairing them with foods high in vitamin C, such as citrus fruits, red bell peppers, strawberries, broccoli, or cabbage. The *Dietary Guidelines* specify that women who may become pregnant should eat foods high in heme iron or consume iron-rich plant foods or iron-fortified foods paired with foods high in vitamin C.

High-Iron Foods
Oysters
Lean red meat or dark poultry meat
Fortified breakfast cereals
Eggs
Spinach
Swiss chard
Baked or refried beans
Prune juice
Raisins

Begin to Improve Your Diet

If following a healthy diet were as easy as it sounds, we would all be perfect eaters. But in fact, even with Americans' interest in diet, weight loss, fitness, and nutrition, very few Americans really follow the advice they are given. There are many reasons why talking the talk is easier than walking the walk. We don't just eat to nourish our bodies; eating fulfills a number of complex psychological and social purposes outside of its nutritional context.

Many women today are health-conscious, but very few follow what could be considered a healthy diet. Fortunately, pregnancy can be an opportunity for change.

With the incentive of giving their children a healthy start in life, many women make considerable changes in their diet while pregnant. If you use the opportunity of your intended pregnancy to really make an effort to eat better, you could help change your habits in the long term and ultimately improve your health.

I would recommend reading through the information about a balanced diet in Chapter 4 for more detailed information on the types of foods that are best for your health. Chapter 9 also has eating tips and recipes that are useful for gearing up for pregnancy. I also encourage you to pay more attention to what you eat day to day and to begin to make these simple changes:

Eat more:

- *Whole grains.* These include bread, pasta, crackers, and other baked goods made with whole wheat flour or other whole-grain flour as the first ingredient, as well as brown rice and other grains such as barley, oats, millet, quinoa, and corn. They have more nutrients and promote a healthier metabolism than refined grains.

- *Fruits and vegetables.* Try to include these at every meal and snack. Include the iron-rich vegetables listed earlier and vitamin C–rich foods.

- *Low-fat, nutrient-rich protein sources.* You will need to boost your protein intake slightly during pregnancy, and it's good to get in the habit of choosing lean meats, low-fat or fat-free dairy products, and protein-rich plant foods such as beans, peas, tofu, nuts, and seeds.

- *Unsaturated fats.* Unsaturated fats are not only good for your heart health, they are critical for your future baby's development. Sources of healthy fats are plant oils such as canola and olive oil, nuts, seeds, soy, and fish. Omega-3 fatty acids, found in fish, omega-3-enriched eggs, some plant oils, and walnuts, may be particularly important for fetal development. Choose lower-mercury fish such as chunk light tuna (not white albacore), shrimp, salmon, pollack, or catfish. Chapter 5 has more information on the mercury content of fish.

Cut back on:

- *Refined grains.* Most baked goods, crackers, and other snack foods, as well as mealtime staples such as pasta and white rice, are made from refined grains, which lack the protein, fiber, and vitamins and minerals of whole grains. They can put stress on your metabolism by causing blood sugar levels to swing wildly.

• *Saturated fats.* These fats are found in animal products such as meat and dairy, and they can have a negative effect on your long-term health by raising your cholesterol levels and your risk of heart disease. Choose lean meats and low-fat or fat-free dairy products to cut back on these fats.

• *Trans fats.* These are fats found in margarine and many processed foods. They help to promote high cholesterol levels, which can lead to clogged arteries and a higher risk of heart disease. Furthermore, these processed fats are not needed by your baby's body and should be avoided during pregnancy. Avoid products that have hydrogenated or partially hydrogenated oils, which are trans fats.

• *Sweetened beverages.* Sodas and other sweetened beverages are a primary source of added sweeteners in our diets, and they have little or no nutritional value. Get out of the habit of drinking any sweetened beverages; reach for water or more nutritious drinks such as whole fruit juice and skim milk.

• *Other added sugars.* Baked goods, sweets, and many processed foods contain added sweeteners that cram calories into the diet without bringing needed nutrients with them. They can also have a roller-coaster effect on your blood sugar levels, which becomes a concern when hormonal changes in pregnancy put you at risk of gestational diabetes.

Reach a Healthy Activity Level

Engaging in regular physical activity can help you get control over your weight, which is important for a healthy pregnancy. Women who are physically fit tend to begin their pregnancies at a healthier weight and are less likely to gain too much weight during pregnancy or fail to lose weight after pregnancy. It's good to engage in some form of exercise regularly—aim for a half hour every day or at least three or four times a week. It can be a structured activity, such as working out at a gym or taking aerobics classes. Or it can be a combination of different activities that are part of an active lifestyle, such as walking or biking around the neighborhood, walking up a few flights of stairs several times at work every day, doing yard work, practicing yoga or Pilates, or lifting free weights at home. Cardiovascular exercise—any activity that raises your heart rate significantly and builds up a sweat—is good for keeping your heart healthy and burning excess calories. Weight lifting and weight-

Make Healthy Foods Convenient

These days we prize convenience, often grabbing snacks and meals on the go. Unfortunately, some of the most convenient foods are also the least healthy, and your best intentions to eat healthier foods can be undermined when you are faced with easier empty-calorie options. When you are at work or out running errands, always bring a healthy snack or two such as a piece of fruit, vegetable slices, low-fat cheese or yogurt, nuts, or whole-grain crackers. You can precut fruits and vegetables and package them in individual bags ahead of time to make them easier to grab on the go. Identify a few healthy food options in the places you frequent—such as the deli that sells fresh fruit, the restaurant with great salads, or the snack machine stocked with yogurt or skim milk. By planning your options ahead of time, you can avoid reaching for those sugary snacks or high-fat foods when you're on the run.

bearing exercises can help you maintain muscle tone and strength. Exercises that build the "core" muscles of your lower back and stomach are great for preparing your body to handle the weight of the fetus in late pregnancy.

Like most things in life, too much exercise can potentially be a bad thing. Athletes who engage in intensely vigorous activity can have fertility problems, especially if they are very lean, and may also have a difficult time gaining enough weight if they try to maintain their activity level during pregnancy.

Address Unhealthy Habits

Habits are hard to break. There are certain habits that are extremely harmful to a fetus and should be stopped completely as soon as you may become pregnant, such as these:

- Smoking
- Drinking alcoholic beverages
- Using recreational drugs or abusing over-the-counter or prescription medicines

You should quit using any of these substances as soon as you begin trying to conceive, because they can potentially cause harm in those early days before you know you are pregnant. While some women have no problem avoiding these substances, those who are addicted to them can have a very difficult time stopping during pregnancy, especially in the throes of new physical or emotional changes that pregnancy can bring. If you have an addiction or suspect you may have trouble avoiding these substances entirely during pregnancy, you should break the habit now and get it under control before even trying to get pregnant. Contact your doctor or the agencies listed in the reference section of this book for help.

If you regularly drink caffeinated beverages, you may want to start cutting back before pregnancy, because you should limit your caffeine intake to the equivalent of one or two cups of coffee per day while pregnant, and because high levels of caffeine may reduce fertility. Unhealthy eating habits, though they may not seem like addictions, can be equally hard to break. That's why it's a great idea to start improving your diet ahead of time and getting used to eating healthier foods while cutting back on sources of empty calories, such as added sugars and fats.

Get Any Medical Conditions Under Control

Certain medical conditions can become more difficult to control during pregnancy. As we discuss in Chapter 5, certain medications are unsafe or have unknown risks during pregnancy. If you are in better health before pregnancy, you are less likely to need medications or have to deal with other medical complications while you are pregnant. Talking with your doctor ahead of time about how to manage problems can help you stay one step ahead of any health problems you may encounter. Metabolic problems—diabetes, high cholesterol, high blood pressure, and obesity—can be exacerbated during pregnancy because of the hormonal changes taking place in your body. Some women even develop metabolic problems only during pregnancy, such as gestational diabetes and pregnancy-induced high blood pressure, or *preeclampsia*. Following a healthy diet may help you prevent these conditions or help you manage them better if they do happen.

Improve Your Fertility with Nutrition

Some women find it easy to get pregnant; others have a harder time. The reasons why some couples are very fertile and some aren't are not fully understood. It's estimated that 15 to 20 percent of couples in the United States have problems with infertility, with higher rates in older couples. Infertility is an equal-opportunity problem: one-third of the time it can be traced to the woman, one-third of the time to the man, and one-third to a combination of factors with both partners. About 80 percent of the time infertility can be traced to a specific cause.

For thousands of years people have speculated on the role food may play in fertility, often believing certain foods make men more potent or women primed for pregnancy. No single food has been found to help make a baby, and most of these ideas are probably myths. However, nutrition can play a role in getting pregnant because:

Polycystic Ovary Syndrome (PCOS)

Polycystic ovary syndrome (PCOS) affects 5 to 10 percent of women of childbearing age. Women with PCOS have many hormonal imbalances, including high levels of male hormones, which can cause acne, excessive hair growth, weight gain, irregular periods, and infertility. The most worrying problem for their long-term health is insulin resistance, in which the body no longer responds to the hormone insulin, which normally helps regulate blood sugar when you eat. When the body is insulin resistant, both the sugar and the insulin build up in the blood.

Eighty percent of women with PCOS are overweight, often with an apple-shaped body type where weight accumulates in the abdomen. The best way to control the effects of PCOS is to lose weight; unfortunately, women with PCOS often have a particularly hard time shedding pounds. Having PCOS during pregnancy puts you at a higher risk of miscarriage, gestational diabetes, high blood pressure during pregnancy, and premature delivery. If you have PCOS, losing a small amount of weight can improve your fertility while also improving your chances of having a healthy pregnancy by bringing your condition under control.

There are medical treatments for PCOS. Birth control pills can help regulate menstrual cycles, improve acne, and lessen male hormone levels, but they don't cure the condition and obviously must be stopped if you want to become pregnant. The diabetes medication metformin can help regulate insulin problems and decrease testosterone production, which can help restore menstrual cycles. The safety of metformin during pregnancy is currently being evaluated. If you have PCOS, your pregnancy will be most successful if you bring your condition under control before pregnancy, through gradual weight loss and possibly medications. Talk with your doctor about the best plan for you.

- Your weight has an important role in your fertility.
- Following a balanced diet contributes to your overall health and fertility.

Weight and Fertility

Weighing too little or too much can affect your fertility. Your body exists in a balance—you take energy into your body in the form of food, and you expend energy through physical activity and the day-to-day maintenance of body organs and tissues. If you constantly eat more than you expend—even by a small number of calories—it can gradually add up to weight gain. Similarly, if you are very active but limit your food intake, your weight will gradually decrease. Collectively, the systems that control your energy balance are called your *metabolism.*

Your metabolic health is intrinsically linked to your reproductive health and your ability to support a pregnancy. A woman's fertility is highly sensitive to the energy balance of her body and the health of her metabolism. The reproductive system "listens" to messages from a woman's metabolism in the form of hormones. When some aspect of metabolism is abnormal, the resulting hormonal changes can affect her fertility and ultimately the health of her pregnancy, because a woman's metabolism controls how nutrients are delivered to her baby.

Women who take in too little energy have reduced fertility. It requires a significant investment of energy to carry a baby to term—an estimated 80,000 calories in total. But a woman's reproductive system is a cautious investor; it doesn't want to invest in a possible pregnancy unless there is a high chance of return. To prove that she has the capacity to nourish a fetus, a woman needs to have a certain amount of energy already in savings in the form of fat tissue. Think of this as your "down payment" on a baby. When a woman has too little fat saved up—usually less than 25 percent of her total body mass—her periods may become irregular, which makes it more difficult to get pregnant. Under about 17 percent body fat, her periods may stop altogether, a condition called *amenorrhea.*

If you are very lean, are an athlete, are rapidly losing weight, or have an eating disorder such as anorexia or bulimia nervosa, you run the risk of not having enough energy stored to support a baby. If your periods are irregular, gradually gaining a small amount of fat tissue may help restore your monthly cycles. Your doctor or a registered dietitian can help you reach a healthier weight while still following a balanced diet with lots of nutrient-rich foods.

The fertility balance is also disrupted when there is too much energy to spare in the form of excess fat accumulation. Women who are overweight or obese can experience irregular periods, decreased fertility, and other reproductive problems. If you are overweight or obese, losing about 10 percent of your body weight can often restore regular menstrual cycles and improve your chances of conceiving. And as we discussed before, your weight loss will also help ensure the health of your child.

Diet and Fertility

While no single food has been shown to improve fertility, following a healthy diet that is filled with nutrient-rich foods may contribute to your overall reproductive and physical health. Unfortunately, there is very little solid evidence about how diet and other lifestyle choices affect fertility—most recommendations are based on small studies or anecdotal evidence.

Some lifestyle choices that have been linked to decreased fertility are smoking, moderate to heavy alcohol consumption, and moderate to high caffeine intake. The problem is that these habits tend to be practiced together by the same individuals, so it is difficult to separate the effects of each one. However, couples in which the female smokes cigarettes have consistently taken longer to conceive in studies. Most larger studies on caffeine intake have found that fertility declines when women's caffeine intake exceeds 250 milligrams per day, about two cups of brewed coffee. The effect of caffeine in each individual is very modest, but considering that 20 percent of Americans consume more than 300 milligrams of caffeine per day, these small effects may add up on a population scale. Drinking more than four alcoholic drinks per week has been associated with delayed conception in a study of 430 Danish couples, and drinking more than eight drinks per week was associated with infertility from ovulatory failure in a study of nearly five thousand women. But another large epidemiologic study found no association between drinking and fertility, so the effect is still unclear.

Because smoking, alcohol consumption, and high caffeine intake are potentially dangerous during pregnancy, the link between these habits and infertility adds yet another reason to cut back before becoming pregnant.

There have been concerns that some foods can affect fertility by influencing hormone levels. Several studies have found that vegetarians have slightly lower levels of estrogen, perhaps because their diets are lower in fat or because compounds in soy-based foods, called *phytoestrogens*, displace the body's natural estrogen. Lower estrogen may lead to decreased fertility in vegetarians, as can a lack of nutrients. A government-conducted study found that very low-fat diets caused women to experience longer menstrual cycles and longer periods, which could theoretically lower their fertility. It is not yet clear how different diets affect fertility, but it's best to avoid any diet that requires you to cut out some of the basic components of a healthy diet. This includes very low-fat, high-protein, or low-carbohydrate diets designed for weight loss.

Male Nutrition and Fertility

Traditionally, women were often blamed when a couple could not conceive, but we now know that men and women are basically equal partners in infertility problems. Male fertility is thought to be declining generally; studies have found that sperm counts are falling worldwide. It has been speculated that environmental factors such as pollutants or pesticides may be contributing to this trend, but no one knows for sure.

Lifestyle factors, including good nutrition, may also have a role in male fertility. Scattered studies have examined the effects of vitamins and minerals—including zinc, magnesium, vitamin C, vitamin E, vitamin D, selenium, and vitamin B_{12}—in improving male fertility. None of these studies points conclusively to one factor that helps improve fertility in men. But collectively they suggest that a healthy diet rich in important nutrients may make a difference. Men can take steps of their own to prepare for pregnancy:

- Eat a diet that is rich in vitamins and minerals, including lots of fruits and vegetables, legumes, whole grains, and lean meats.

- Follow the advice in Chapter 4 of this book for improving your intake of healthy fats while lowering your intake of unhealthy saturated and trans fats, which may lower sperm count.

- Take a multivitamin/multimineral supplement daily to make up for any possible deficiencies. But don't overdo it: taking a large dose of any one nutrient won't do anything to improve your chances of pregnancy and could be harmful to your health.

- Adopt some healthy habits, such as quitting smoking, reducing alcohol consumption, managing stress levels, and staying active.

Although following a well-nourished diet is an important part of your reproductive health and fertility, nutrition is only part of the fertility picture. As I mentioned before, the majority of fertility problems can be traced to a specific cause, and some problems can be medically treated. If you and your partner are concerned about infertility, see your doctor.

Planning for Pregnancy: The Bottom Line

While many women have perfectly healthy unplanned pregnancies, if you have the opportunity to plan ahead, you have a better chance of entering pregnancy in the best possible health and will have an easier time adjusting to your pregnancy. See this time—whether it is a matter of weeks, months, or years—as a "prep course" for pregnancy. I encourage you to read through the entire book to learn about all the things you can do to make your pregnancy a healthy one. Then you can start identifying any changes that you may need to make. The following checklist (adapted from Brigham and Women's Hospital Department of Nutrition patient education material) will help you figure out if you are nutritionally ready for pregnancy. If you can agree with all the statements, you are well on your way:

- I maintain a healthy weight—either in the "normal" range of the BMI chart or as close to that range as I can be while still nourishing my body. My weight is not fluctuating greatly, and I'm not overeating or dieting.
- I have been taking a folic acid supplement alone or as part of a daily prenatal multivitamin.
- I eat a variety of nourishing foods every day. The majority of the foods I eat are vegetables, fruits, whole grains, legumes, low-fat or fat-free dairy products, lean meat, poultry, and fish.
- I choose healthy unsaturated fats over saturated fats, and I avoid products with trans fats.
- I consume sweets in moderation and cut back on added sugars, refined grain products, and sweetened drinks.
- I have cut back on caffeine, I have stopped drinking alcoholic beverages, and I don't smoke or take recreational drugs.
- I have discussed pregnancy with my doctor and have talked about how to manage any preexisting medical conditions.

2

How Pregnancy Works

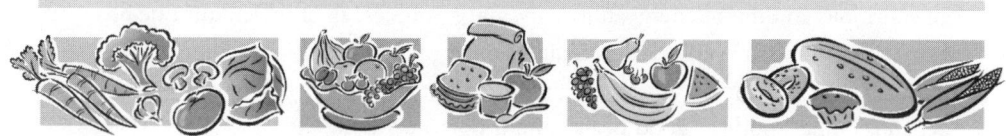

Pregnancy is surely the most astounding process that the human body can undergo. That a woman's body can support the development of another human being from a single cell to a newborn is truly a marvel. We still do not understand all the intricacies of pregnancy, in terms of both fetal development and a mother's ability to adapt to and provide for a fetus.

Advice for pregnant women can easily start to sound like a very boring to-do list: do this but don't do that; eat this but avoid that. It can all seem very dry and disconnected from the strange and amazing events unfolding inside your body. The purpose of this book is not to simply tell you what to do; I'm hoping to also help you understand what is happening inside your body and why nutrition is so important during pregnancy. In doing so I hope to make my case stronger and more compelling than a simple to-do list, and I also hope to satisfy some of your natural curiosity about your pregnancy.

What It Takes to Make a Baby

During pregnancy, a single cell grows and transforms to become a human baby. All of the complex actions that must be performed to carry out this feat are programmed right into the baby's genetic material—her DNA contains the basic instructions to divide her cells; to form different kinds of tissues and then different organs; to orient body parts in the correct position; to form complex networks to carry blood, air, nerve impulses, and hormones throughout the body; and to grow a brain that will be able to quickly sense her environment and learn new information when she is born.

But the instructions are no use without the physical ingredients needed to build a human body. Though genetics play an enormous role in development, genes are not the only factor at play. Building a baby from a single cell requires marshaling an enormous amount of energy, nutrients, and resources, all of which must be provided by the mother's body. It also requires the right conditions—a protected environment, free from toxic substances or injury. At every stage of pregnancy, a baby depends on her mother's good health and proper nutrition.

Your body provides a steady supply of nutrients—carbohydrates in the form of glucose for energy, proteins and fats to build the structures of the body, and vitamins and minerals to carry out key processes in cells. All of the components needed to build a baby come from the mother's body. Some of these nutrients might come from stores your body keeps, reserves of energy or other elements that are tucked inside your tissues. But most of the nutrients you pass on to your baby come from what is circulating right in your blood. And the contents of your blood vary according to what you eat every day. That's why many women find they must make significant changes in their diets while they are pregnant. You're no longer choosing foods just to fill you up, stay healthy, or provide pleasure for yourself. You're also choosing the raw materials that will nourish your baby into life.

During the early part of a baby's development in the womb, his cells are rapidly dividing and laying a blueprint for later growth, a basic outline for all the organ systems of the body. Later, the cells that form these organs begin to swell, increasing the overall size of the fetus. Growth reaches its briskest pace in the second and third trimesters, as the blueprint gets fleshed out into a more developed body. Information about pregnancy often focuses on either the mother or the child. You've probably seen drawings of the different stages of a fetus's development inside its mother's womb, and you've probably also heard about the changes that take place in your body throughout your pregnancy. It's easy to lose sight of the fact that pregnancy is essentially a relationship between two beings: a woman and her growing baby. A woman's body is not simply a passive receptacle for a fetus. At every stage, pregnancy is a series of complex interactions between a woman's body and her baby. This relationship is the basis for understanding why nutrition matters in pregnancy.

Table 2.1 shows how your baby's body changes throughout pregnancy. Your baby's progress—and the changes in your body—are detailed in the next section.

The First Trimester: Laying the Foundation

The first couple of weeks of your pregnancy probably happen without you knowing about it. Your baby begins his journey as a single cell called a zygote, which means "yoked together" in Greek. This is the cell that results from the fusion of a sperm and egg. About thirty hours after it forms, the zygote divides, making two cells where there was one. Those two cells split again, making four, and four become eight. After a few of these cell divisions, the blastocyst, as it is now called, contains one hundred or so cells and has traveled from its origin in your fallopian tubes and entered your uterus.

During this time, the ball of cells relies on a wash of fluid from its mother's uterus to provide needed nutrients. But eventually it must establish a more direct connection to its mother if it will survive. At this point the blastocyst divides into distinct layers. An inner ball of cells will eventually become a baby. A thin swath of cells around the outside will become the placenta that serves as a direct link between your bloodstream and your child's. Even in the early stages of this process, the nutrients available in your body have an impact on your baby's health.

A few days after fertilization, the tiny blastocyst attaches to the walls of its mother's uterus and digs in—it actually invades its mother's tissue and burrows out its own little bunker there. The outer layer of cells around the blastocyst form fingers of tissue that burrow between the layers of its mothers tissue. These cells wander through the tissue until they reach their mother's blood vessels, where they are able to access nutrients from her bloodstream. Meanwhile, a cavity forms between the inner cells, which are destined to become the baby, and the outer cells. This cavity, called the amniotic sac, eventually surrounds the whole embryo and fills with fluid. The baby is then exposed to its environment only through the umbilical cord, which carries two arteries and one vein that are connected to the placenta.

The lining of your uterus undergoes changes during this time, and the tissue becomes swollen and filled with nutrients for the embryo. This lining, called the decidua, will become your side of the placenta, a large mass of tissue that serves as a central hub for exchanging nutrients and waste between you and baby. Around this time you will miss a period and may begin to notice the earliest signs of pregnancy, such as tender breasts.

Table 2.1　Your Baby's Progress

EMBRYONIC OR FETAL AGE (WEEKS)	LENGTH	DEVELOPMENTAL CHANGES	BODY SHAPE
1	0.1 mm	Blastocyst implants in walls of uterus.	
3	1.0 mm	Early spinal cord and gut develop.	
4 to 5	2.0–3.0 mm	Arm and leg buds form.	
6	1.5 cm	Heartbeat can be detected with ultrasound.	
8	3.7 cm*	Eyelids and ear canals form; head becomes more rounded; muscles grow, allowing small movements.	
12	8.8 cm*	Body is more elongated; sex can be distinguished externally; hair and nails grow.	
16	14.0 cm*	Head is held erect; lower limbs are more developed; movements can be felt.	
24	32.0 cm	Body is longer but very lean; alveoli (air sacs) in lungs form.	

Table 2.1   Your Baby's Progress *(continued)*

EMBRYONIC OR FETAL AGE (WEEKS)	LENGTH	DEVELOPMENTAL CHANGES	BODY SHAPE
28	38.5 cm	Brain forms its characteristic folds; eyelids open; testes descend in boys.	
32	43.5 cm	Body fat begins to accumulate; toenails form.	
36	47.5 cm	Nails have grown to fingertips; body is plump.	
38	50.0 cm	Brain cells become more efficient; chest grows more prominent.	

*Early fetal lengths are measured from the top of the head to the rump, because legs are not fully developed enough to measure accurately from head to foot.

The time after implantation to about eight weeks after an egg is fertilized is called the embryonic period. It's a time of laying the foundations for later growth, as the dividing cells begin to form specific tissues and then those tissues begin to form distinct organs. The embryo, which until now has depended mostly on fluids and surrounding tissues in your body for nutrients, now gets its supplies from the burgeoning placenta, which is composed of both your cells and your baby's.

In the fourth week, the embryo is a mere C-shaped cylinder. The nervous system is the first to form, and the region that will become the brain begins to enlarge. The heart also starts beating during this week, and arm and leg buds appear. The cells of the embryo have organized themselves into three layers: an inner layer will become the internal organs such as the liver, lungs, intestines, stomach, and urinary tract; the middle layer will become heart, blood vessels, bones, muscles, and reproductive organs; and the outer layer will become the nervous system and skin. In the next weeks, the embryo, which is still just a few centimeters long, begins to grow a distinct head with a jaw and facial features, and limbs with webbed fingers and the buds of toes.

At the end of eight weeks, the embryo is called a fetus. All of its major organs, body systems, and external features have at least begun forming by this time, but they still have a long way to go to grow and mature. In this time, growth has been relatively slow while the blueprint of the baby's body is laid out. Your baby is still just a few inches from head to foot. After two months, growth takes off, and a mother's nutrition is important for fueling this growth. Teeth and fingernails begin to grow, and arms lengthen to their final proportions. By twelve weeks, the external genitalia are visible, giving a clue to the baby's sex.

Your Body in the First Trimester

During the first three months of pregnancy, your body undergoes radical changes to adjust to the new life it now supports. Even though the later stages of pregnancy appear more dramatic to the outside world, the first months will most likely bring the most dramatic internal changes for you. Imagine that your body, with all its cells, tissues, and organs, is like a city. This city has developed systems to transport supplies, food, and consumer goods to each neighborhood and to transport waste and other products out of the city. Every system in place has been developed around the needs of the city's population. Now, imagine that the population of the city suddenly jumped, by the equivalent of a small town. Suddenly transportation systems need to be rerouted, roads must be built, sewage systems need to be extended—major changes must occur to accommodate this new growth. Your body must accomplish a similar task during pregnancy. Every system of your body changes to accommodate the new life growing within you.

How does your body "know" to make these changes? Most of them happen in response to hormones, chemical signals that can either act locally between two tissues or can be sent through the bloodstream to distant sites in the body. The first signs of pregnancy are a result of the hormone human chorionic gonadotropin, or hCG (this is the hormone that pregnancy tests detect), as well as elevated levels of estrogen and progesterone. By about a month into your pregnancy, you will probably begin to experience the first symptoms—nausea (morning sickness isn't just a

The Amazing Placenta

The placenta is a pancake-shaped organ that carries nutrients from mother to child and waste from the baby out to mother to be removed from her body. Your blood and your baby's don't come in direct contact—even tiny oxygen molecules must travel through five layers of tissue to reach your baby's bloodstream. Although both you and your baby contribute tissue to the placenta, it is mostly made of cells and blood vessels that were created by your fetus. It is stuffed with tiny fingers of tissue called villi that are filled with blood vessels; together these branches create a large surface area for the exchange of nutrients. The placenta requires extra energy and nutrients to grow. It thickens until about four months into pregnancy, when it starts to stretch further around the baby, eventually covering about one-third of the surface of your uterus.

The placenta is much more than a passive cargo carrier. A growing fetus has specific needs; it doesn't just take nutrients from its mother as they come. The placenta acts as a manager of this transport, matching the needs of the fetus with the nutrients available from the mother. Some small nutrients, such as oxygen, carbon dioxide, and salts, diffuse easily back and forth between mother's and child's tissues. Other nutrients, such as glucose, lactate, and amino acids—the major sources of energy needed for a fetus to grow—must be shuttled across cell membranes by special carriers, and some require energy to move them back and forth. The placenta is also responsible for sending out hormones that stimulate changes throughout your body. It helps protect the fetus from certain infections, and it even helps to protect against your own immune system, which otherwise might try to attack the baby as a foreign invader. The placenta even functions as a "radiator" keeping the baby warm. With all of these duties, the placenta requires a good deal of energy on its own—half or more of the extra energy and oxygen that are delivered to a woman's uterus late in pregnancy are used to support the placenta! Humans would never have developed such an energy-guzzling system unless the placenta was performing some extremely important work.

All the nutrients you give your baby pass through your placenta first. So fetal nutrition doesn't depend just on what you eat; it depends on having a good delivery system. Not every aspect of fetal nutrition is under your control. The size and efficiency of the placenta play a big role in how well a fetus thrives, and these properties are largely controlled by genetics. However, there is some evidence that the state of a mother's nutrition and whether she is over- or underweight may influence the growth of the placenta. One of the important research questions that has not been answered about pregnancy, in fact, is to what extent a woman can improve her fetus's nutrition through her own behavior and to what extent it is out of her control.

morning event; it may strike any time of the day), vomiting, a frequent need to urinate, and changes in food preferences. Several weeks into your pregnancy, the volume of your blood will begin to increase, especially the clear fluid called plasma that surrounds your blood cells. Your blood volume may grow by one-third to one-half of its normal level, to better supply the growing baby and placenta. Your heart rate increases as your heart begins to pump more blood, and the muscle mass in your heart even increases. Some of these changes may leave you feeling dizzy or fatigued. The dramatic changes in hormone levels during pregnancy may cause your emotions to swing more wildly. Your breasts may enlarge and continue to feel tender or even tingly, and your nipples may darken.

The Second Trimester: Growing and Growing

While the essential blueprint for the baby's body was laid down in the earliest part of pregnancy, the second trimester is mostly a time of building. During the fourth month, growth actually slows slightly, but it soon picks up again and moves quickly. Your baby's body doubles in length in the fifth month, and by month six she has achieved 60 percent of her birth length and 20 percent of her birth weight. All of this growth is made possible by nutrients shuttled from your blood to your baby's through your placenta. At the same time, the gross features that formed in the first trimester continue to become refined. Facial features become more distinct. The soft skeleton hardens, and muscles develop, allowing your baby to move around more. Air passages in the lungs finish branching, and the lungs prepare to take in oxygen. By twenty weeks, the body has reached more normal proportions. The legs reach their final relative position, and you may begin to feel your baby's movements.

Your Body in the Second Trimester

Now that your body has made the major adaptations needed to accommodate a fetus, you may find that the symptoms of pregnancy are less severe in the second trimester. But as your baby grows, your body must make room. Your intestines are the first organs to get shifted around to make room for baby. The expanding volume of your blood may cause nosebleeds, tender gums that bleed easily, and headaches. You should be especially vigilant about the health of your teeth and gums, because pregnant women are more prone to developing gingivitis. The growth of new blood vessels into the pelvic area may also heighten sexual arousal.

Some women find that their skin becomes blotchy and darker in certain places, a symptom that usually goes away after pregnancy. You will now also begin feeling the effects of the baby's weight. Your own body weight will rise as your fat stores increase, and you may need to adjust your posture to accommodate the weight in your tummy. You may experience backaches, cramps, swollen legs and ankles, and varicose veins.

The Third Trimester: Preparing for Life Outside

In the third trimester, your baby prepares to leave the safety of your womb and enter the real world. During these last months, muscle and fat tissue are laid down over the newly formed organs, and the skin surrounding it all grows thicker. Brain cells, which were produced abundantly in early fetal life, now begin to organize themselves into the more complex structures of the brain. The lungs prepare to breathe air, and the nervous system initiates rhythmic breathing movements. The baby begins to follow cycles of sleeping and wakefulness. The eyes open and gain the ability to sense light. Your baby continues to grow, and his arms and legs are flexed against your body, which is becoming ever more crowded.

Your Body in the Third Trimester

Instead of all those subtle effects of hormones that you felt at the beginning of pregnancy, in the third trimester your body is adjusting to the sheer size of the baby inside you. Your uterus now extends almost to your liver, and your internal organs are getting squeezed. That can create digestive discomfort, heartburn, increased need to urinate, and back pain. During this time you are gaining weight steadily, which is a critical part of a healthy pregnancy that we'll spend time discussing. You will feel easily fatigued, and the weight and size of your baby make certain movements difficult. Eventually you will begin to experience the contractions in your uterus that signal it is time to give birth.

Understanding Fetal Nutrition

In the next chapter, I'll discuss some exciting new research that has been changing the way we think about fetal development and health. More and more, scientists

A Baby's First Home

In addition to providing direct nutrients to a growing baby, your body also gives him a home and a protected place during this important time. Your uterus expands fifteen times its initial volume over the course of pregnancy. Amniotic fluid bathes your baby, providing a watery cushion that protects against shocks and pressure from the outer environment. Surrounded by fluid, a fetus is essentially weightless. At the same time, he has enough freedom of movement to move against the walls of the uterus and the amniotic sac, helping the newly forming limbs to exercise. He also receives physical stimulation as you move throughout the day, and he experiences the patterns of sleeping and wakefulness of your body. Your baby is always kept warm by the heat of your body. He will hear muted sounds from outside but is mostly surrounded by the rhythmic sounds of your own blood flowing. In essence, the uterus is a place of physical protection from the outside world but one that allows enough stimulation to help the fetus develop.

While the womb is a protected place, it is not shut off from the world. Many potentially harmful substances and conditions can enter a baby's first home. Chemicals you breathe or ingest, radiation you are exposed to, extreme temperatures, physical injury, too little or too much of a particular component of your diet—all of these factors can potentially affect your baby. We'll discuss potentially harmful habits and substances later in this book. The most important thing you can do to care for your baby before he is born is to care for your physical and emotional well-being. Caring for yourself will help ensure that your body is the best home it can be.

are finding that the kind of environment a person experiences in the womb, including good nutrition, may have a profound impact on later health. But by now this shouldn't come as a surprise. As you've seen, at every stage of pregnancy, a fetus depends completely on its mother for nutrients and a protective environment. Some of the factors that create this environment are controlled by genetics, but others depend on a mother's behavior and diet. Pregnancy is a relationship between mother and child, and there are ways that you can take action to ensure that relationship is a healthy one.

The term *fetal nutrition* may be new to you. After all, when we think of nutrition we think of eating food. Fetuses don't "eat" in the traditional sense, but their mothers do, so we focus on maternal nutrition during pregnancy, and we don't think about a child's nutrition until after birth. But it's important to remember that nutrition is a critical part of the health and development of a fetus. In fact, the time a baby spends in the womb is in many ways the most critical time to receive good nutrition. Nutrition actually plays a larger role in determining growth before birth than it does after birth. Once a baby is born, good nutrition is necessary for healthy growth, but how large a child grows is for the most part a matter of genetics. In contrast, in fetal life nutrition and the health of the mother are most important in determining how well a baby grows.

During pregnancy, your baby needs energy to grow. Just like children and adults, fetuses need three major components of nutrition: carbohydrates, fats, and proteins. We get these nutrients by breaking down food; fetuses receive these nutrients directly from their mother's blood, already broken down into a simple form. Fetuses also need vitamins and minerals to carry out functions in their bodies and assure that their organs develop to their full size, so their requirements for some of these components are different from those of a grown adult. That's why your diet should reflect the needs of your baby as well as your own.

Not every part of a baby's body develops at the same time. Development is a piecemeal process. The nervous system, for instance, develops in the early embryo before any other system. A baby's intestines and bladder are essentially fully formed at birth, but other parts of the body may take years to fully develop and mature in a child. That's why certain nutrients may be especially important at certain stages of life, such as folic acid in the first couple weeks of life and calcium in adolescence.

Your Health in Pregnancy: The Bottom Line

While we talk a lot about what a baby needs as it develops in the womb, the recommendations in this book are designed to help you, too. A common refrain in pregnancy is that "nature favors the baby." In some ways, a developing fetus behaves a bit like a parasite, taking resources from its "host," the mother. This is not a criticism of pregnancy but a simple fact: at times, a mother and her fetus are in a kind of competition for nutrients—especially when nutrients are in short supply—and often the fetus wins out. Poor nutrition during pregnancy can adversely affect a mother more than it would at other times of her life. For instance, if you consume too little calcium, the mineral may be leached from your bones to provide for the needs of your baby. Your body's reaction to a limited dietary supply of a nutrient is often to deplete your own internal stores. Many of the recommendations given to pregnant women (such as to consume lots of calcium) are important for your own health as well as the health of your unborn child.

3

Why Fetal Health
Lasts a Lifetime

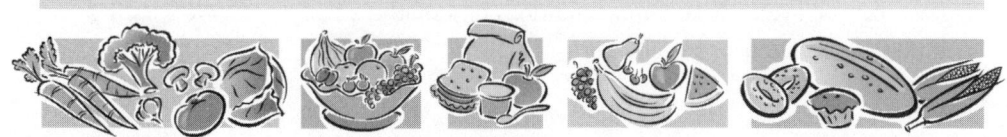

We've long believed that a mother's health habits are important during pregnancy. But research from the past two decades has shown that good nutrition in pregnancy may be even more critical than was once thought. Evidence is building that nutrition during fetal life has lasting effects on a person's health, metabolism, and risk of developing chronic disease later in life. This research shows that your health during pregnancy not only helps you deliver a healthy baby but will also help your baby grow to become a healthy adult.

This area of research is still very new, but several insights are beginning to emerge from it:

- Poor nutrition in fetal life can predispose a person to develop chronic disease as an adult.
- Conditions in the womb can permanently alter a baby's metabolism.
- Taking care of your body by eating a balanced diet, maintaining a healthy weight, and managing any health problems *before* and *during* pregnancy are important for both a healthy delivery and your baby's long-term health.

These findings reinforce what we've already known: good nutrition matters for a healthy pregnancy (see Figure 3.1). They also suggest that good health in the earliest stages of life will have lifelong benefits. In this chapter, I hope to give you a broad overview of recent research into how fetal nutrition affects adult health. It points to one basic message: health in the womb forms the foundation for health later in life.

Your body is much more than simply a home for your baby as she develops. During the time you are pregnant, your body and the nutrition you provide your baby will actively shape her, as a sculptor shapes clay. This phenomenon has been called "fetal programming." Fetal programming is a new field of scientific research that has stirred interest in the importance of good nutrition in pregnancy. It suggests that the overall health and conditions of a mother's body can leave a lasting impression on her baby's health.

Metabolism and Health

To understand why nutrition has such a crucial impact on health and disease, its important to understand the concept of a healthy metabolism. Every year, your body takes in about one thousand pounds of food, and you replace almost every molecule inside your body with a new one. Most of the tissues of your body are constantly being torn down and reconstructed, all powered by energy from food. Your metabolism includes all the systems and chemical reactions in your body that

Figure 3.1   Health Effects of Fetal and Early Childhood Nutrition

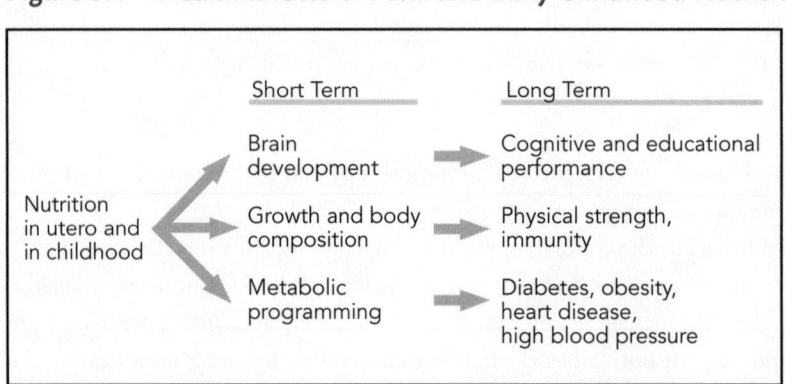

are responsible for turning food into energy for the body, turning energy into new tissues, storing extra energy in reserve, expending energy, and disposing of waste products. It is basically the collective engine that keeps you alive. Many of the primary causes of death and disease in developed countries stem from metabolic "engine problems," including heart disease, diabetes, and obesity. Many of these problems are caused by misuse of our metabolisms—driving our engines improperly with poor diet or letting them languish with a sedentary lifestyle.

We have long recognized that events during fetal development can affect a child's health. For instance, if something happened to prevent a fetus's brain from developing properly, it could result in permanent brain damage. During fetal life, a baby's metabolic engine is assembled just like other parts of the body such as the brain. If something interferes with the development of the metabolic engine, it may have an impact on how that engine runs throughout the child's life.

While we've always known that events during development could lead to physical or mental health problems, it has only recently been accepted that the same process could apply to a person's metabolism. Instead, if a man developed heart disease or diabetes, we used to assume that he may have inherited a genetic predisposition to the disease (a bad engine) from his parents or that he probably followed an unhealthy lifestyle or poor diet (improper engine maintenance).

Current research shows that another factor may come into play. The predisposition to disease may have come during development—an engine assembly problem. It is only in the past couple of decades that scientists have recognized the role that fetal life, infancy, and childhood have in establishing a healthy metabolism. We now understand that disease is a cumulative process of all your experiences. It includes the genetic "parts" you were given; how those parts were assembled during fetal life, infancy and childhood; and how you take care of them throughout your entire life.

The good news about this view is that each stage of life represents an opportunity to prevent disease and improve lifelong health. This is often called the "life course" approach to health and disease. Certain stages of life are more critical than others, and different aspects of health have different critical periods when we can best intervene.

The Origins of Fetal Programming

The interest in fetal programming began in the late 1980s when a British epidemiologist named David Barker began noticing something odd: he found that areas of Britain that had high rates of infant mortality also had higher rates of death from heart disease. Why was this so strange? Typically we think of heart disease as an unfortunate by-product of a prosperous life—eating too much food, consuming lots of saturated fat, and living a sedentary lifestyle. But infant mortality is generally higher in areas that are poorer, where life is more difficult and rich food more scarce. Barker and his colleagues found another paradox when they looked at records from a large group of men born in Hertfordshire, England, in the early part of the 1900s. The researchers found that men who had been very small at birth or one year of age were more likely to have died from heart disease as adults. For instance, those who weighed eighteen pounds or less at one year had almost three times the rate of death from heart disease as those who weighed twenty-seven pounds or more. Those who were small in early life but became overweight later on were at the highest risk for heart disease. Barker suggested that poor nutrition in early life somehow makes the body more susceptible to the effects of an affluent diet.

Barker's studies brought about a new wave of research into the area of fetal development and disease. In addition to the link between birth weight and cardiovascular disease, many studies have shown that other health problems have been linked to birth weight, including high blood pressure, obesity and overweight, and diabetes.

All of these diseases result from problems with the metabolic engine. These studies suggest that poor nutrition in the womb can cause lasting changes to the metabolism of a fetus and can affect how that child's metabolism functions in adulthood. They also suggest that a mother's health during pregnancy might affect the way her baby was built—could "program" her baby's body to function in a particular way. The idea has been called fetal programming, the Barker hypothesis, or, more recently, the developmental origins of adult disease. What seemed radical about these new studies was the idea that a characteristic at the very beginning of life could somehow determine one's health near the end of life.

Barker's findings found many skeptics, who pointed out that the associations he found were so remote in time from each other that many other factors might explain them. However, the association between low weight at birth and cardiovascular disease was also found in other populations in the United States, India, Sweden, and South Wales. As part of the Nurses' Health Study, Harvard researchers examined health information in a group of more than seventy thousand women and found a strong relationship between birth weight and risk of cardiovascular disease. Once the results were reproduced several times, it became harder to ignore them.

Further research into fetal programming has shown that our health can be "imprinted" into our bodies as we are developing. A striking example of the influence of fetal nutrition on adult health comes from babies who were born during the Dutch Hunger Winter, a famine that occurred in World War II. Near the end of that war, a strike called by the Dutch resistance as part of an Allied campaign resulted in Germans halting shipments of food into Holland. A severe winter and little food led to a brief but severe famine in the region, with daily food allowances as low as 300 to 600 calories per person, which represents just one-eighth to one-fourth of the typical recommended caloric intake for a pregnant woman. The

What Birth Size Means

What does it mean to be born small or large? Some babies are born smaller simply because they are born earlier. The longer a baby stays in the womb, the larger he will grow. The final weeks of pregnancy are a time when the body is becoming fuller, plumper, and heavier as fat and muscle are added, and premature babies do not spend as long undergoing these processes in the womb.

But some babies are born small for the relative amount of time they spent in the womb. The size and weight a fetus reaches depends on its environment: how big its mother's uterus can stretch to accommodate it, the nutrition it receives, the hormones it is exposed to. If a fetus's growth is restricted by any of these factors, it will be born small but later will often grow faster to "catch up" to its genetically determined height. These babies who are "small for gestational age" seem to be the ones who are particularly programmed for increased disease risk in later life. For classifications of birth size, see Figure 3.2.

Though the initial studies in fetal programming focused on babies who were born small, poor health is also seen with babies born too large. Large babies have been shown to have higher rates of obesity and diabetes later in life, and they can also create complications for delivery. Eating well and gaining the recommended weight during pregnancy (see Chapter 7) will help ensure that your baby is born at a healthy weight.

Figure 3.2   Growth Chart

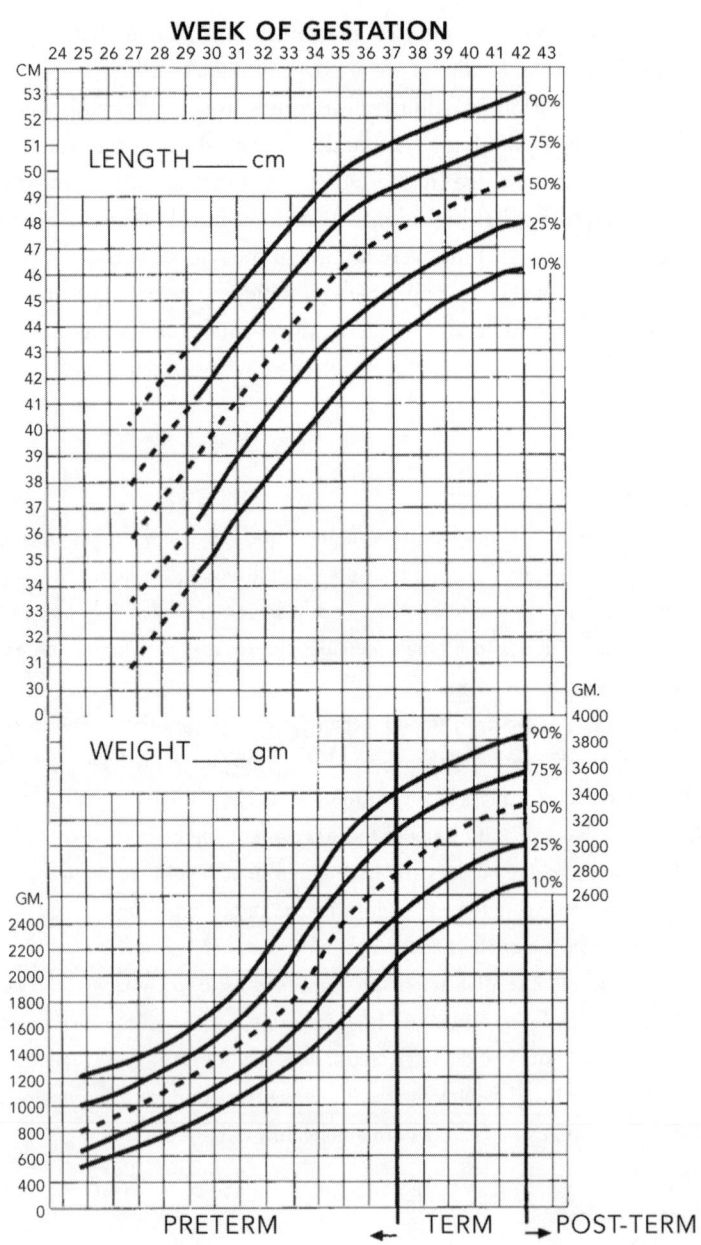

infants who were conceived or born during this time grew into adults who had a higher incidence of glucose intolerance—a condition that precedes diabetes—as well as higher rates of coronary artery disease and high blood pressure.

People who were small at birth but gained weight the fastest after birth or became overweight adults were at greatest risk of disease compared with those born just before or after the famine. This idea is also somewhat counterintuitive. If a baby is born very small, most of us would instinctively want to feed that baby more to encourage her to grow to a normal size. But these studies suggested that this kind of "catch-up" growth is the worst thing for a baby. The environment in the womb is not the only important factor for our later health; instead, the interplay between our health before and after birth somehow determines our predisposition to developing disease.

Disease Can Be a Result of Incorrect Planning

Why would a person who develops under conditions of deprivation have more serious health problems later in a lifestyle of comfort? One explanation is that diseases such as heart disease and diabetes can occur when the environment turns out to be different from what was predicted during development.

Imagine putting together the "engine" of the metabolism. If you were concerned about a shortage of fuel for your engine, you would design it to be very fuel efficient. But if fuel is plentiful, you might not bother—you might even design it to burn through fuel quickly to keep it running faster. The same may be true for our metabolism. Those babies who developed during a famine may have been preparing to face a world where fuel—in this case food—was scarce. Researchers Peter Gluckman and Mark Hanson have called this phenomenon "predictive adapted responses." A fetus, they argue, has ways of sensing its environment and using that information to match its metabolism to the conditions it predicts it will meet in the world. If it is deprived of needed nutrients in its mother's womb, it adjusts its body's systems to compensate. In other words, maybe those babies who developed during a famine were "programmed" to be fuel efficient. When they were born, and the famine ended, their bodies were less equipped to handle the much more comfortable lifestyle in store for them—for instance, their metabolism might store the extra fuel they got from a rich diet rather than burning off the calories.

The Thrifty Hypothesis

The human body has evolved ways of surviving in difficult conditions, but these survival strategies may actually backfire when they confront a more luxurious lifestyle. This idea is often called the "thrifty hypothesis." Many researchers now think that the human body has evolved mechanisms to make its metabolic engine more fuel efficient. Our ancestors survived best when they could weather out periods of starvation and food scarcity. But now that we are faced with an entirely different environment—an overabundance of food—those fuel efficiency mechanisms can actually cause disease. We respond to our environment by storing extra fuel (obesity), losing our ability to process incoming fuel properly (diabetes), and eventually allowing by-products of metabolic reactions build up in our systems (atherosclerosis and heart disease). Some of these fuel efficiency mechanisms are built into our genes—often called the "thrifty genotype." Others may be acquired during our development in our mother's womb—called the "thrifty phenotype." Once we better understand these factors, we can help our children and ourselves avoid falling into a lifestyle that works against our basic biology.

How Programming Works

How does a person's body become "programmed" during development? In other words, how do nutrition and other environmental conditions get translated into differences in how a person's body behaves?

• *A mother's nutrition and metabolism affect her baby.* A woman's body is not simply a receptacle for her growing baby. It plays an active role in determining how the baby's body will develop and function in the outside world. The nutrition your baby receives is influenced by your diet, how big your placenta grows and how well it functions, how large your uterus can grow, the levels of hormones circulating in your bloodstream, and how much you weigh. While some of these factors are genetic, many are at least partially controlled by your metabolic health. While your baby is growing inside you, she depends on the efficiency of *your* metabolic engine to deliver the nutrients she needs to grow. There is a clear connection between poor nutrition in mothers and a higher risk of metabolic disease in their children. These health problems can arise when mothers are undernourished, but they also can develop if mothers have health conditions that stem from *over*nourishment, such as obesity and diabetes. Being in good metabolic health helps a mother deliver good nutrition for her baby, which helps ensure her baby's metabolism is assembled in the healthiest possible way.

• *Small changes early can lead to big differences later.* The essential concept of programming is that small disturbances early in life can result in big problems later because of the way the body develops. During development, a blueprint is laid out very early for different organ systems. Even when the embryo is just the size of a seed, all of the major organ systems have already been assigned a place in the tiny body—it's now just a matter of cells dividing, growing, and becoming more and more specialized and complex. Because the early stages set the foundation for all later stages, they are especially sensitive to change or insults. Like a fundamental flaw in a building's foundation, these changes could cause problems that are widespread.

• *Programming can change how organs form.* One of the ways that programming probably happens is by altering how specific organs grow and develop. We can see evidence of this in animals. If a fetus is undernourished, its body might divert resources to critical areas such as the brain, while other parts of the body get short shrift. To all appearances, a baby born with smaller organs would seem perfectly normal, but the effects might appear later in life in the form of poor health or disease.

• *Timing matters.* As we discussed in Chapter 2, the development of a fetus doesn't progress smoothly and steadily. The nervous, digestive, respiratory, circulatory, and reproductive systems all follow their own timetable of development. Each of these systems has a "critical window" of time in which your nutrition and the baby's environment can affect their outcome. The piecemeal development of the human body means that different stages of life will be more critical for different aspects of the body. For instance, folic acid is one of the most essential vitamins for pregnant women, because it is needed to complete a critical stage in the development of the nervous system. But this event occurs very early in pregnancy, before many women know they are pregnant. That's why we recommend that all women of childbearing age get a good supply of folic acid before they become pregnant.

- *People respond to their environments differently.* Some people seem to eat what they like without their health ever suffering. Other people are predisposed to storing fat or developing metabolic problems. Many aspects of our metabolism are set by the time we are born, and these programmed responses interact with our environment and our lifestyle to determine our health. Each of us needs to respect the unique way our body functions. Trying to overfeed a small baby will only work against the baby's natural programming. Babies should be fed healthy foods according to their appetites and be allowed to grow as they were programmed to do.

Putting the Hypothesis to the Test

The Barker hypothesis is, as its name states, just a hypothesis at this point. It has generated a lot of interest but also quite a bit of controversy. How much of this can you believe? When the first studies came out, they showed an intriguing association in human populations. Since that time, many more studies have been conducted, and animal studies have begun to document specific effects in a fetus that occur in response to changes in its nutrition. All of this offers some pretty convincing evidence that fetal programming is a reality.

One of the open questions about fetal programming relates to scale. Many of the studies that have shown a clear effect on programming from extreme conditions: women who were pregnant during a famine, animals that were fed very low-calorie or low-protein diets, babies whose growth was severely restricted in the womb. But the extent to which a more subtle shortfall in calories, proteins, or specific nutrients might affect fetal development is less clear. Not every baby whose growth is restricted in utero goes on to develop diabetes, high blood pressure, or heart disease. In many ways, it is a testament to the remarkable flexibility of human development that healthy babies are born under so many varied conditions.

Further research should help elucidate which aspects of fetal programming are the most critical for health and may point to interventions we can take to prevent disease. Whatever the specifics turn out to be, fetal programming and the Barker hypothesis have changed our entire way of thinking about how to keep people healthy. The diseases we have been talking about may be termed "lifestyle diseases" because they are often brought about by our own behaviors—eating too much, eating the wrong kinds of foods, engaging in sedentary activities. We already know ways to help prevent these diseases in adulthood by following good diet and exercise habits and a healthier lifestyle. The Barker hypothesis implies that we should also focus on the very *beginning* of life to have an impact on disease. And people who may be predisposed to certain diseases because of their early life experiences can take special measures to follow healthy habits throughout their lives.

While fetal programming offers a radical new perspective on the origins of disease, little of the research has been translated into specific advice for pregnant women. The kind of scientific consensus needed to make broad recommendations for the public often takes years or decades to gather. On one hand this slowness is frustrating for parents who want answers now. But on the other hand, this process helps protect you from getting advice that's premature, exaggerated, or just plain wrong.

What Does Fetal Programming Mean for You?

We don't yet know the best ways to prevent some of the problems that occur in fetal life, and further research is needed to tease out the details of the fetal origins of adult disease. But there are a few clear implications that emerge from these findings.

• *Good health starts early.* The fetal period is an important time for establishing good health in your child. Strong evidence shows that the fetus is extremely sensitive to harm and that the changes that take place in development may have long-term effects. Other research is also looking at how nutrition during infancy and early childhood also affects later health, so once your baby is born you should continue to make good nutrition a priority. Many scientists are now advocating a life course approach to preventing disease. They view health as a continuum in which there are certain critical periods for susceptibility to poor health, including the period of fetal development. Instead of focusing on disease prevention only in middle age, we need to begin to think of the long-term health of our children from the beginning of life.

• *Healthy mothers have healthier babies.* We've always known that some behaviors by a pregnant woman—such as drinking alcoholic beverages, taking certain drugs, or eating a diet that lacks key nutrients—can have lasting effects on the unborn baby. But fetal programming shows that a variety of environmental conditions such as poor nutrition, stress, or poverty could potentially alter the course of fetal development and put a person at risk for poor health.

Try to achieve the best health you can *before* pregnancy, including reaching a healthy weight and eating a nourishing diet. The time before and throughout pregnancy is a perfect opportunity to adopt healthy behaviors that support the success of your pregnancy and provide a good environment for your baby's development. It's not just about a grocery list of things to eat; it's a matter of a healthy overall metabolism: maintaining a healthy weight; eating enough food to support you and your baby; eating a balanced diet with the right proportion of protein, fats, and carbohydrates; getting enough vitamins and minerals, especially ones that are needed in key stages of fetal development. Keeping fit and lowering stress levels can also affect your body and the environment you create for your child during pregnancy.

The steps you take to stay healthy now can be a model for keeping yourself healthy after pregnancy and an inspiration for other family members. The following chapters will offer you advice on how to achieve the best nutrition during pregnancy. The insights that have come from fetal programming research show us why following these guidelines is even more important than was once thought.

Is Fetal Programming a Threat to Mothers?

I'd like to address some of the concerns that expectant mothers may have when they hear about fetal programming research. It's easy for information about fetal programming in the media to sound threatening to moms. Many women already feel as if their health habits are under scrutiny—by their partners, family, coworkers, and even perfect strangers—when they are pregnant. If more and more attention is paid to the importance of fetal life in overall health, will it lead women to blame themselves for their children's health problems, or will society cast more blame and scrutiny on mothers? The Barker hypothesis is often introduced in the media with a catchphrase such as: "Blame your health on your mother," or something equally provocative.

My hope is that we will use the information we learn about fetal health for the better. I don't think that women should be scared or threatened by any of the current research in fetal programming. Instead, I hope that women will look positively on the opportunity they have to use this information to have healthier pregnancies. I hope that we as a society will respond to these new ideas by ensuring that women have access to the resources and services they need to stay as healthy as possible before, during, and after pregnancy. I hope the information will lead to a better understanding about how our behavior and environment cause poor health and disease, because many nutritional health problems are linked to larger factors such as economic and social status, mental health, stress, and ethnic and racial background. And I hope that, ultimately, this research will benefit women's health by reminding us that healthy mothers are the foundation of a healthy population. Remember, the best thing you can do for your baby is to keep yourself healthy, and that means taking care of and valuing your own well-being.

Fetal Programming: The Bottom Line

Your metabolism is like your body's engine. Your metabolic health depends on how your engine is designed genetically, how it is put together in the womb, and how you take care of it throughout your life. And remember:

- Recent research has shown that aspects of a person's metabolism are "programmed" in the womb as the metabolic engine is being assembled.
- The effects of fetal programming can influence adult health, changing a person's chance of experiencing later health problems and chronic disease.
- Taking special care of your health and diet during pregnancy can help ensure that your baby is born healthy and grows into a healthy adult.

4

Eating Well for
Your Baby-to-Be

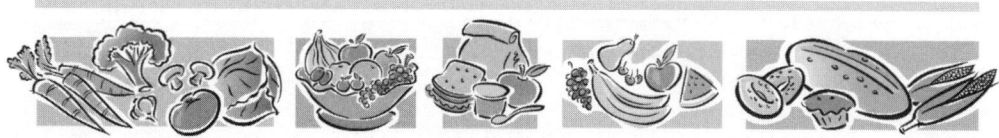

By now I hope I've convinced you that your nutrition matters during pregnancy and that the careful choices you make to follow a healthy diet now will not only help you deliver a healthy baby but will help ensure your child's health throughout life. This time deserves a special emphasis on good nutrition, even if it means restraining yourself from a few indulgences or breaking a few dietary routines.

You've probably heard the maxim that you are "eating for two" during pregnancy. It's a confusing message. The phrase is often taken to refer to the *amount* of food you eat. In reality, pregnant women who are well nourished to begin with don't have to eat too many more calories than they normally do. Even in the stages when your baby is growing the fastest, you need to eat only an extra 300 calories every day—that's the equivalent of a bagel, an egg with toast, or a banana with a large glass of milk. This may translate into an extra snack every day, or it may mean that you can eat slightly larger portions at meals than you're used to.

For most women, the most important focus of pregnancy is not increasing the *quantity* of what they eat but raising the *quality*. It's all too easy to pad your diet with food that fills you up and tastes good but doesn't provide the nutrients that you need to support the growth and development of your child.

What is a healthy diet for a pregnant woman? A healthy diet should accomplish a few things:

- Provide enough energy (calories) to support your body and the growth of your baby's body
- Provide all the raw materials (proteins, fats, vitamins, and minerals) needed to keep your body healthy and construct your baby's body
- Avoid or limit foods and other substances that have negative effects on your baby's body
- Support your overall metabolic health by allowing you to maintain a healthy weight, blood sugar level, and blood pressure

Making Real Changes for Your Health

For many women, the time when they are pregnant may be the first time they really begin to seriously evaluate the healthfulness of their diet. With a baby growing inside them, they suddenly become aware of the nutrients in their food and whether that food is nourishing or is simply a source of empty calories. Many women go to considerable effort to change their behaviors and eating habits while they are pregnant—but what happens afterward?

You can use the time when you are pregnant to make real, lasting changes in your eating patterns that will help you stay healthier after pregnancy, reducing your risk of developing chronic disease later in life. Many mothers are concerned about the weight they gain during pregnancy, especially in the midst of caring for a newborn. The effort you make to change habits now can put you in a better position to lose weight safely and keep your body healthy after pregnancy. Some of the advice in this book is pregnancy-specific, especially the sections about specific nutrients that pregnant women need. But much of the information about eating a balanced diet and making healthier food choices applies to all diets; what is healthy for your baby is also healthy for you. Changing dietary habits is a difficult task. But with the incentive of your baby's health, you can put the process in motion. The final chapter of this book will discuss diet after pregnancy and will give you tips on incorporating the hard work you've done while pregnant into your daily life.

Pregnant women can understandably feel overwhelmed by advice about nutrition. Too often, we hear about all the foods that are "bad" to eat during pregnancy, and this can leave some women feeling as if there is nothing they can eat. There is no need to feel overly constrained by a rigid diet during pregnancy, and, with the exception of some important harmful substances, there are few foods that should be banned during this time. In fact, I'm going to save a discussion about all the things that should be "out" during pregnancy for the next chapter. In this chapter, I'd like to talk about improving your diet so that the nutrition you provide yourself and your baby is the best it can be. It's not just about saying no to certain things; it's about saying yes to healthy, nutritious foods. Rather than looking at each food you eat as either good or bad, we'll look at how the foods you eat on a daily or weekly basis add up to a healthy diet. I am not going to give you a complicated plan that you must follow while pregnant, as some books do, because such a strict set of rules simply isn't supported by science. Instead, to ensure your diet is optimal you need to understand and follow only a few simple steps:

- Pay special care to a few key nutrients that babies need to grow.
- Choose foods that maximize important nutrients and limit empty calories.
- Eat a balanced diet.

Special Needs in Pregnancy

Your body has special needs for certain nutrients during pregnancy. Many of these can be covered by eating a balanced diet with healthy foods. But some may require boosting your intake of certain foods during pregnancy. And some are difficult to cover by diet alone—we'll discuss supplements briefly here and in greater depth in Chapter 6.

Calories

As I mentioned before, your energy requirements are slightly higher during pregnancy. This energy is used for your baby's growth, to construct your placenta and new blood vessels and other tissues, and to power the metabolism of these new tissues. And because the average woman increases her body mass by 20 percent during pregnancy, every movement she makes requires 20 percent more energy by the end of her term. But unfortunately, your need for calories is not a license to overeat. Your body needs about 80,000 additional calories during your entire pregnancy. That amounts to about 300 extra calories a day, the size of a substantial snack. It may be difficult to tell if you are adding this number of calories to your diet, because most of us have no idea how many calories we consume from day to day. Use your hunger as a guide in the short term, and monitor your weight gain over the long term to help gauge whether you are eating the right number of calories (Chapter 7 will explain your weight goals in detail). Repeated bouts of nausea or dramatic changes in food cravings and aversions can be an obstacle for consuming enough calories. If you find it difficult to eat as much as you need, you may need to seek help from a doctor or nutritionist to find ways to stay nourished.

Protein

You need more protein during pregnancy than at other times in your life, because proteins provide the building blocks of growing fetal tissues. Pregnant women need about 70 grams of protein per day, which is 25 grams more than usual, the equivalent of adding a portion of meat or a large glass of milk to your usual diet. However, the majority of Americans get more than enough protein in their diet. If you tend to load up on high-carbohydrate foods, such as breads and pasta, and don't often eat meat, tofu, beans, or dairy products, you need to make a special effort to eat high-protein foods. Otherwise, simply make sure that you are eating some protein with every meal and most snacks. Adding an additional protein-rich snack to your regular diet is an easy way to cover both the extra calories and protein needed during pregnancy.

Folate (Folic Acid)

In 1998, folate was added to all enriched cereals and grain products in the United States to raise the levels of folate in the diet of the entire population. This vitamin plays an important role in the development of an embryo. Women with low levels of folate in the diet have an increased risk of having babies with neural tube defects such as spina bifada, a condition that arises when the tiny tube of tissue destined to become the brain and spinal cord fails to seal properly in the early development of an embryo. In Chapter 1, we talked about the importance of taking folate *before* becoming pregnant. The closing of an embryo's neural tube occurs very early in pregnancy, before some women are even aware they are pregnant. However, women who are already pregnant should continue to take folate, because low levels also seem to increase the risk of complications during pregnancy. The federal *Dietary Guidelines* call for women who are pregnant or of childbearing age to consume folic acid through supplements as well as natural food sources. Folic acid supplementation of about 600 micrograms per day is advised for all pregnant women, as is eating foods that are naturally high in folate, including orange juice, spinach, asparagus, kale, collard greens, cooked dried beans and peas, and whole-grain breads and cereals.

Folic Acid in Foods
Daily goal: 600 micrograms (includes amount in prenatal vitamins or supplement)

1 cup of most breakfast cereals (some are higher, such as Total, with 400 micrograms)	100 micrograms
½ cup boiled lentils	180 micrograms
½ cup pinto beans	147 micrograms
½ cup boiled asparagus (six spears)	130 micrograms
½ cup boiled spinach	130 micrograms
½ cup wheat germ	100 micrograms
½ cup orange juice, from frozen concentrate	109 micrograms

Iron

With too little iron in the diet, the body is unable to produce enough hemoglobin, the molecule that enables red blood cells to carry oxygen to the body's tissues. Studies have found that low iron levels in pregnant women are associated with an increased risk that their babies will be born early and underweight. And having too little iron puts you at risk for anemia and fatigue, which is especially common in pregnancy, as your blood dilutes to expand in volume. Pregnant women need double their usual recommended daily dose of iron to grow and support the placenta, which is rich in blood vessels. Iron can be found in red meat, dark meat from poultry, and some dark leafy green vegetables. However, it can be difficult for most women to get enough iron from foods. Many pregnant women need to take an iron supplement of around 30 milligrams per day throughout pregnancy. We'll talk about choosing a prenatal supplement in more detail in Chapter 6. Even with a supplement, you can still benefit by eating iron-rich foods. The iron found in enriched cereals and vegetables such as spinach is not as easy for the body to use as that found in animal products; you can help improve the absorption of the iron you eat by pairing iron-rich foods with fruits and vegetables containing vitamin C.

Iron in Foods

Daily goal: 30 milligrams (Most women need help from a supplement to make this goal.)

3.5 ounces extra-lean hamburger	3.14 milligrams
1 cup dry roasted mixed nuts	5.07 milligrams
1 egg	0.73 milligrams
1 cup boiled soybeans	8.84 milligrams
1 cup General Mills Total breakfast cereal	22.4 milligrams
1 cup Kellogg's Raisin Bran	4.6 milligrams
1 packet Quaker Instant Oatmeal	6.3 milligrams
½ cup boiled spinach	3.2 milligrams

Zinc

Several studies have found that women who have low levels of zinc in their diet are at a higher risk for preterm delivery and a baby with a low birth weight. Clinical trials of zinc supplements have not yielded any clear-cut results showing a benefit to taking extra zinc, but it's a good idea to consume higher levels of this mineral during pregnancy. Zinc can be found in animal products, especially red meat, and also in whole grains, nuts, legumes, and some fortified breakfast cereals. Most women do not need a special zinc supplement, but you might benefit from taking one (about 25 milligrams per day) if you have an illness or are generally in poor health or under stress, because these conditions can interfere with your body's ability to deliver zinc to your baby.

Zinc in Foods

Daily goal: 15 milligrams

1 cup canned baked beans	4.24 milligrams
1 3-ounce extra-lean hamburger patty	5.4 milligrams

¼ cup sunflower seeds	1.7 milligrams
1 cup cooked peas	2.0 milligrams
8-ounce container plain nonfat yogurt	2.0 milligrams
½ cup boiled spinach	0.7 milligrams

Calcium

A fetus collects about 25 to 30 grams of calcium from its mother over the course of a pregnancy, mostly during the third trimester. Most of this calcium is used to fashion bones and cartilage, but part of it also helps blood vessels contract and dilate, nerves transmit signals to one another, muscles contract, and glands secrete hormones.

However, most of this calcium is provided by mom free of charge. A woman's body becomes amazingly efficient at absorbing and using calcium during this time, creating a surplus that is saved for her baby. In fact, adding extra calcium in the diet does little to add to the amount available to a fetus. But it's still important for your own health to make sure you are getting enough calcium in your diet, about 1,000 milligrams per day; otherwise, you body may divert calcium from your bones and teeth to nourish your baby, compromising your own health. Several studies have suggested that calcium may also help to offset the risk for preeclampsia—a condition characterized by swelling, high blood pressure, and protein in the urine—especially among women at risk for the condition. If you consume a lot of dairy products, on the order of three servings of milk, cheese, or yogurt a day, supplements aren't necessary, but if not you could benefit from taking a calcium supplement. Adolescent or young mothers, whose bones are still growing, should try to get even more calcium, about 1,300 milligrams every day. These women should take a calcium supplement—otherwise, they may be putting their own growth at risk as well. Calcium needs are greatest in the last trimester of pregnancy, but it's recommended that you keep this level up throughout your entire pregnancy.

Calcium in Foods
Daily goal: 1,000 milligrams (1,300 milligrams for women under eighteen)

1 cup yogurt	350–400 milligrams
1 cup milk	300 milligrams
1 ounce cheese	200 milligrams
1 cup cottage cheese	150 milligrams

1 cup firm tofu	200 milligrams
¼ cup almonds	75 milligrams
½ cup broccoli	50 milligrams

Vitamin C

Unlike calcium, the amount of vitamin C made available to a fetus depends on a mother's diet. Vitamin C is an antioxidant that protects the body's tissues from damage and is needed to build collagen and chemical signals in the brain. Too little vitamin C can result in pregnancy complications such as premature birth and infections. Pregnant women should consume about 10 milligrams per day more than other women, or 85 milligrams a day total. You can easily reach this amount by eating fruits and vegetables every day, especially citrus fruits, broccoli, bell peppers, strawberries, and tomatoes. Vitamin C–rich foods also help you better absorb the iron in your diet. If you decide to take a supplement, don't overdo it; many people have developed a habit of popping vitamin C pills under the mistaken impression that it will ease a cold. Too high a dose of any vitamin could put your baby in danger.

Vitamin C in Foods
Daily goal: 85 milligrams

½ cup sweet red bell peppers	100 milligrams
½ cup sweet green bell peppers	56 milligrams
1 baked potato with skin	20 milligrams
1 orange	70 milligrams
1 cup diced tomatoes	23 milligrams
1 mango	57 milligrams
½ cup cooked broccoli	50 milligrams
1 cup raw strawberries	85 milligrams

Vitamin A

Vitamin A is critical in many functions of the body, including vision, immune function, and the growth and development of the early embryo. A deficiency of vitamin A during pregnancy is associated with growth restriction of the fetus, preterm

Teenage Pregnancies

Adolescents and teenagers who become pregnant have special dietary needs because their own bodies are not yet fully developed even as they are supporting the growth of a fetus. Studies on adolescent pregnancy have shown that young mothers and their fetuses are in competition for nutrients, more so than adult mothers. And adolescents have twice the likelihood of having a baby of low birth weight or having a preterm delivery. Any deficiency in the diet could compromise the health of mother or baby. Even though a healthy diet is even more important for younger pregnant women, adolescents often have poorer dietary habits than adult women and may need to make more radical changes in their eating patterns to have a healthy pregnancy. And because more than 90 percent of teenage pregnancies are unplanned, teens are far less likely to be prepared for pregnancy. Adolescents and young women can benefit greatly from seeking early prenatal care, including a nutritional assessment that can help them to make the dietary changes they need.

Pregnant teens need extra calcium and phosphorous, both of which are important for bone health, as well as slightly greater amounts of magnesium and zinc. They should aim for extra servings of low-fat and fat-free dairy products, as well as lean red meat, leafy green vegetables, whole grains, and legumes. Taking a prenatal multivitamin can also help safeguard the diet of a young mother (see Chapter 6 for more on supplements). But young women also shouldn't overdose on vitamin or mineral supplements, particularly vitamin A, which can build up in the body and become toxic to a fetus.

birth, and low birth weight, all of which can cause short- and long-term problems for a baby's health. At the same time, taking very high doses of vitamin A through supplements has been shown to cause birth defects. While it's fine to get some extra vitamin A through a prenatal multivitamin, I would recommend seeking your extra vitamin A through foods rather than supplements. Vitamin A is found in many fruits and vegetables in the form of carotenoids, such as beta-carotene, the pigment that gives carrots, winter squash, mangoes, and sweet potatoes their orange color. Beta-carotene is also plentiful in leafy green vegetables. The high levels of beta-carotene in these foods do not result in excessive levels of vitamin A in the body. Preformed vitamin A is found in animal products such as meat, eggs, and dairy, and is generally not concentrated enough to cause toxicity.

Vitamin A in Foods
Daily goal: 2,565 I.U.

½ sweet potato, with skin	2,310 I.U.
½ cup raw carrots	1,089 I.U.
1 cup green leaf lettuce	660 I.U.
1 cup skim milk with added vitamin A	495 I.U.
1 large egg	264 I.U.
½ cup cooked frozen collard greens	1,617 I.U.
1 cup Cheerios	495 I.U.

Make Food Choices That Maximize Nutrients

Your main goal during pregnancy is to ensure that your diet is filled with all the components needed to support your baby. That means maximizing the nutrients in the foods you eat and making sure they are nourishing rather than just empty sources of calories. We can divide the types of foods you eat into general categories that are probably familiar to you: breads and grains, fruits and vegetables, protein foods, and dairy products. We'll talk about how to put them all together into a balanced diet. But first, how do you choose the foods within each group that are healthiest for you and your baby?

Breads and Grain Products

The grain group is the primary source of carbohydrates in our diet and includes everything from rice, pasta, cereal, and bread to chips, cake, and cookies. A healthy diet should include as much as possible foods made from whole grains rather than refined grains. What's so great about whole grains? Most of the carbohydrates you eat are broken down or converted to sugars, which are the body's main source of energy. The digested sugars are absorbed into your bloodstream. Your body then pumps out insulin, a hormone that tells the tissues in your body that food is on the way, and they absorb the sugar from your blood to use for fuel. Carbohydrates that are easily digested cause your blood sugar and insulin levels to spike and then drop again as the sugar is quickly absorbed. Over time, severe ups and downs of blood

Vegetarian and Special Diets

Pregnant women should take a conservative approach to their diet. We don't always know how special diets affect growing fetuses and whether or not they will lack important nutrients needed to support a pregnancy. *Never* try to follow a diet that requires you to eat certain foods exclusively, such as high-protein or high-carbohydrate diets. Your baby needs a balanced diet that includes carbohydrates, fats, and proteins.

Vegetarian women may have a difficult time meeting their protein needs if they are not careful to include a wide variety of protein sources in their diet. It's not just the *amount* of protein that is important. The *kind* of protein you eat also matters, because proteins are made up of different combinations of amino acids, and vegetable sources sometimes lack the certain amino acids that animals like us need.

It is possible to achieve your protein needs on a vegetarian diet with some special effort, though some vegetarian women choose to eat meat during the time of pregnancy just to be safe. Those who continue with their usual diet should aim to eat lots of protein-rich legumes (beans, lentils, chickpeas, soybeans/tofu), whole grains, nuts, seeds, and, if lacto-ovo vegetarian (eating eggs and dairy), dairy products such as milk, cheeses, and yogurt. Don't rely on one kind of food for your protein. The best way to cover your bases is to eat a wide variety of different plant foods. Make sure you have one or more protein-rich food at *every* meal and snack.

Women who are vegan (do not eat eggs or dairy products) may want to consider changing their diet during pregnancy for the sake of their baby's health. If they continue to follow a vegan diet, they should consult a registered dietitian to plan a diet that will best cover their needs and follow the recommendations closely.

If you don't eat much meat or dairy, or are vegetarian, you may need to supplement your diet with a few important nutrients. Vitamin B_{12} is found largely in animal products and is needed by a fetus to grow new cells. Vegetarians may need to take a B_{12} supplement, either alone or as part of a multivitamin. Vitamin D is usually added to milk and is also produced by the body with sunlight exposure. People who do not eat dairy, especially those who do not get much sun exposure, could also use an extra dose of vitamin D of 10 micrograms (400 I.U.). You also may be at risk for iron and zinc deficiency—see Chapter 6 for information about prenatal supplements. I would recommend that every vegetarian or vegan woman talk with her doctor or a registered dietitian about nutrition during pregnancy.

sugar levels can lead the insulin signaling process to fail, resulting in chronically high blood sugar levels, or diabetes. Pregnant women are particularly susceptible to developing diabetes, and unhealthy blood sugar levels may have long-term effects on your baby's metabolism and health. Carbohydrates that take longer to digest—such as whole-grain foods—have a more moderating effect on your blood sugar. The 2005 *Dietary Guidelines for Americans* developed by the federal government now recognize whole grains as one of the key types of foods to boost in the diet.

Fiber is a type of carbohydrate that cannot be broken down into sugars, so it passes through the digestive system largely undigested. Even though it is not a source of energy, fiber has some important benefits for health. It helps to moderate the rise and fall of blood sugar, in part because the fiber in your foods helps to slow the digestion process down, preventing other carbohydrates from being converted to blood sugar too quickly. It also helps prevent constipation, one of the most common digestive complaints during pregnancy. In the long term, eating plenty of fiber-rich grains may help you maintain a healthy weight, because fiber keeps you feeling fuller longer. And fiber can help to lower blood cholesterol levels by trapping cholesterol-rich bile acids in the digestive system and preventing the cholesterol from being absorbed.

To get the healthiest form of carbohydrates, make these food choices as much as possible:

• *Choose products made from whole wheat instead of refined wheat flour.* The vast majority of grain products on the market are made with refined wheat flour, or white flour, which is made by removing the portions of the wheat grain that contain vitamins and fiber, leaving only simple carbohydrates. White bread is digested in the body similarly to pure sugar. More and more, you can find whole-wheat products such as bread, crackers, cereals, pasta, tortillas, and pita, which are more nutritious and gentler on your blood sugar. Make sure that "whole wheat flour" is the first ingredient—some products are made with "wheat flour," but unless it's whole, it's just plain old refined white flour. Also look for the fiber content on the label, and choose foods that are higher in fiber.

• *Try other whole grains.* White rice undergoes a similar refinement process to wheat, removing a great source of fiber, B vitamins, and other nutrients. Choose brown rice over white. And other whole grains, such as barley, millet, corn, quinoa, or buckwheat, can add fiber, protein, and nutrients to your diet—plus add some interesting variety to your meals.

• *Limit heavily sweetened foods.* One of the primary sources of carbohydrates in our diet is added sweeteners such as high-fructose corn syrup. Sweeteners are added to many processed foods and baked goods and can be found even in foods you wouldn't think of as sweet. Get in the habit of checking labels for added sweeteners. Be aware that many may be disguised to sound healthier by using terms we associate with whole grains and fruits, such as brown rice syrup, pectin, fruit syrup, and fruit concentrates. It's fine to include a few sweet things in your diet, but the bulk of your carbohydrates should come from whole grains, fruits, and vegetables, not sweeteners.

• *Add up the sugar.* Check the total sugar content in the nutrition label of your foods. The "sugar" category includes naturally occurring sugars, such as the lactose in milk, so it can't tell you how much of the sugar comes from added sweeteners. But you can use this number to compare similar products to find ones that are less sweet.

• *Avoid unhealthy fats.* Many grain products are made with fats that are unhealthy (see the next section). When choosing crackers, breads, chips, and other baked goods, look for products that are free of hydrogenated oils.

Making the Most of Fats

You may think of a healthy diet as one that is very low in fat. But that's not entirely true. There is a place for healthy fats, and in fact, fats are necessary for your baby's body to grow and develop. Some fats are necessary for our bodies to function. The problem is that—similar to the added sweeteners that clog up our diet with simple sugars—too much fat often takes the place of other nutrients in the diet. (The current *Dietary Guidelines* recommend that adults keep fat intake to 20 to 35 percent of total calories.) Different kinds of fats have different effects in the body; most of the excess fat we eat is particularly bad for us.

Recent research has shown that choosing healthy fats over unhealthy fats can make a difference in long-term health and help adults avoid heart disease. But good fats are particularly important during pregnancy. The fats you eat are broken down and carried in your bloodstream. While the transfer of fats from mother to fetus is a complicated process, the type of fat your fetus receives depends on what's in your diet. You should strive to fill your diet with the fats your baby needs to grow rather than fats that are useless or even detrimental to health.

Saturated fats raise the level of "bad" (low-density lipoprotein—LDL) cholesterol in the blood and are associated with higher rates of heart attacks and strokes. These fats are found in animal products such as meat and dairy and in a few plant sources such as coconut. They are also added to baked goods and many processed foods to make them taste richer. You should limit the level of saturated fat in your diet by choosing low-fat dairy products and lean meats and by using vegetable oil instead of butter in cooking.

Trans fats are made by altering vegetable oils so that they can remain solid at room temperature, a process called hydrogenation. They are found in most margarines and many manufactured foods, especially baked goods such as cookies and crackers and chips. Trans fats are particularly bad for health because they not only raise LDL cholesterol but also lower the amount of "good" (high-density lipoprotein—HDL) cholesterol in the blood. Trans fats are known to cross the placenta and make their way into fetal tissues. Because these are manufactured fats, their effect on development is unknown. Some studies have shown that the presence of trans fats in the umbilical cord—and indication of a maternal diet high in trans fats—was associated with lower amounts of healthy fats. Trans fats should be avoided as much as possible during pregnancy.

Unsaturated fats, which include monounsaturated and polyunsaturated fats, are found in fish, plant oils, nuts, legumes, and seeds. These fats have been shown to have a beneficial effect on cholesterol levels in the blood. They also contain essential fatty acids, which are fats that are needed for your fetus to grow but can't be manufactured in the body. Included in this category are omega-3 fatty acids such as docosahexaenoic acid (DHA), which recent research suggests may be particularly important during pregnancy. The best sources of DHA are fish, omega-3-enriched eggs, and some plant oils, such as walnut oil. But as we'll discuss in the following chapter, eating too much fish may possess some danger for your fetus. Fish oil pills or DHA supplements may be an alternative, and we'll talk about how to choose the best ones in Chapter 6.

So changing your diet to boost good fats while limiting bad fats can help ensure your baby's health—and your own. Here is a healthy strategy for fat in the diet:

- Limit the saturated fat in your foods while choosing unsaturated fats instead.
- Cook with plant oils such as olive oil instead of butter or lard.
- Boost your omega-3 fatty acids with plant oils, some fish (see Chapter 5 for guidelines on mercury and fish), and a fish oil or DHA supplement.
- Eat low-fat versions of foods that are typically high in saturated fat such as meat and dairy.

- Avoid any product with hydrogenated or partially hydrogenated vegetable oils in the ingredient list—these are trans fats, and they're found in many processed foods. The FDA is moving toward requiring products to list the level of trans fats. Until then, many trans fat–free foods will also voluntarily list trans fats on their labels and are labeled as trans fat free or free of partially hydrogenated oils.

Protein Foods

Protein foods include meat and animal products, as well as protein-rich plant foods such as legumes, nuts, and seeds. As I mentioned before, protein is a critical nutrient during pregnancy. To get the healthiest sources of protein, follow these tips as much as possible:

- *Aim for complete proteins.* Every protein is made of a set of building blocks called amino acids. We need certain amino acids from our diet in order to construct new proteins. Animal proteins provide us with all the amino acids we need; these are called complete proteins. Plant foods do not provide a complete set of amino acids, so to get all the amino acids you need from a plant-based diet, you need to eat a variety of different protein foods and may need to eat more protein than someone who eats meat and dairy. Because providing your baby with the necessary protein is so important, it's good to eat meat, fish, chicken, and dairy products while you are pregnant (see sidebar on vegetarian diets during pregnancy).

- *Watch out for saturated fat.* Meat, dairy, and other animal products are sources of saturated fats, which you should keep to a minimum. To maximize the good nutrients in your diet while limiting the unhealthier ones, choose the leanest cuts of meat and fat-free or low-fat dairy products. Eggs are also fine in moderation. Fish is a great source of unsaturated fat as well as complete protein, but because of human pollutants that find their way into fish, pregnant women need to be particularly careful about the fish they eat. See Chapter 5 for more details.

- *Eat plant proteins to add nutrients.* While animal foods offer the most complete and efficient sources of protein, varying the protein you eat with plant foods can also add some other important nutrients into your diet. Beans, soybeans, nuts, seeds, peas, grains, and other protein-rich plant foods often contain unsaturated fats, vitamins and minerals, and fiber.

Dairy Products

Dairy products are good sources of calcium and protein, both of which are needed during pregnancy. To make the healthiest choices from the dairy group, follow these tips as much as possible:

• *Choose low-fat and fat-free foods.* Dairy products are a prominent source of unhealthy saturated fat. Whenever you have an option to use fat-free or low-fat options, do so. They will have just as much protein and calcium as the higher-fat versions.

• *Limit added sweeteners.* Many dairy products such as ice cream, yogurt, and flavored milks come with a load of added sweeteners. Choosing these foods is better than simply eating candy or other empty-calorie foods, but to make them healthier, look for unsweetened or low-sugar options and try adding fruit, vanilla, or other less sweet flavors. For a discussion on the use of artificial sweeteners in pregnancy, see Chapter 5.

Fruits and Vegetables

There are few people who couldn't benefit from eating additional fruits and vegetables, especially pregnant women. All fruits and vegetables are worthy additions to your diet, but are some better than others? The important strategy for pregnancy is to choose foods that give you a wide range of vitamins and minerals and are especially rich in the ones you need.

• *Go for variety.* Fruits and vegetables are loaded with vitamins, minerals, fiber, water, and other nutrients that are great for your baby's health. The best way to take advantage of the nutrition they offer is to eat a wide variety of different kinds. A simple way to add variety is to mix colors; the pigments that give fruits and vegetables their color also provide different nutrients. And a varied palette also makes meals more visually appealing.

• *Choose whole fruits and vegetables.* Whole fruits and vegetables provide fiber and more nutrients than juices and other processed foods. Fill your diet with whole fruits and vegetables as much as possible. Frozen foods are fine, as are canned (but look for canned fruits that are packed in juice or water, not syrup, and canned vegetables that are lower in salt).

   • *Include vitamin C–rich fruits and vegetables every day.* These include citrus fruits, bell peppers, strawberries, kiwi, cantaloupe, broccoli, and tomatoes.

   • *Include dark leafy green vegetables every day.* These power vegetables contain vitamin A, which many pregnant women are deficient in, plus folate, iron, and other

Fluids and Beverages

Staying hydrated during pregnancy will help your body deliver nutrients to your baby and will also help prevent constipation and fatigue caused by dehydration. Keep a bottle of water handy throughout the day to help keep you hydrated. Drinking water is also important if you are vomiting or having diarrhea, and in general it can help keep you feel well if you are having stomach troubles.

For beverages other than water, try to put your drinks to work for you. Choose nutritious drinks that add protein, vitamins, and minerals, rather than just sugar. Skim milk is a wonderful beverage during pregnancy; it has plenty of protein and calcium and not too many calories, and it helps keep you hydrated. Drinking whole fruit juices and fruit smoothies are also a great way to add nutrients with your water. Fruit smoothies that include the whole fruit also add some fiber, which is something that regular juice lacks. See Chapter 9 for some smoothie and drink ideas. Avoid beverages that provide empty calories such as sodas, sweetened fruit drinks, punches, and "-ades." Many fruit drinks have only minimal juice and plenty of sweeteners; 100 percent fruit juice is a better choice.

Keep caffeine to a minimum by choosing beverages that are caffeine free or lower in caffeine, such as decaffeinated tea. If you drink a lot of diet sodas, you may want to limit your intake during pregnancy to cut down on artificial sweeteners and caffeine. See Chapter 5 for more information.

Be aware that caloric beverages are foods, too, and many of them have quite a lot of calories. They should be included as part of your total caloric intake for the day. It's easy to sip a high-calorie beverage as if it's water, but doing so can contribute to excessive weight gain.

needed vitamins and minerals. Examples include spinach, collard greens, bok choy, Swiss chard, romaine lettuce, and kale.

Making healthier food choices is easiest when you have control over what goes into your meals. Americans are getting more and more of their foods from restaurants than ever before. And even when we buy foods from the grocery store, many of them are processed foods and prepared meals. In order to appeal to our tastes (and get us to buy more), prepared foods and meals are often stuffed with unhealthy fats and sugars and are low on real nourishment. Making healthier choices doesn't mean you can't eat out or cook a frozen meal now and then. But you will be most successful if you choose more whole foods that you prepare yourself. Fresh whole foods can be fast, too. It just requires a bit more thought and creativity to put foods together in simple and appealing ways. Chapter 9 provides some specific recipes and snack ideas that make delicious use of healthier food choices. Try these out, and you may develop an appreciation for foods you don't have to guess the ingredients of. There are also tips for choosing wisely when you are eating out.

The Beauty of Balance

When I told you that eating a balanced diet is one of the most important steps you can take during pregnancy, it probably didn't sound like earth-shattering science. We hear the command to "eat a balanced diet" so many times that few of us stop to think about what it means. It may sound simple, but following a balanced diet is actually not an easy task, and it's one that few Americans accomplish.

Different people may have vastly different ideas of what kinds of foods are "healthy," perceptions that are influenced by our education, our peers, the books and magazines we read, and the advertisements all around us. But whatever foods we think are good for us—whether it's tofu, certain vegetables, organic cereals, or foods with added vitamins and minerals—we tend to believe that a healthy diet just means eating these foods. But including a few healthy foods in your diet doesn't add up to *balance*.

Balance isn't about the individual foods in your diet; it's about the way you put them together. It's important to look at the *proportion of calories* that come from different food groups. By eating the healthy choices from each food group and eating the right proportion of foods from each group, you will be helping to make a broad range of different nutrients available for your baby (see Table 4.1).

Table 4.1 A Healthy Balance

FOOD GROUP	NUMBER OF SERVINGS PER DAY	SERVING SIZE
Breads and grains	6–11	Smaller than you think: 1 slice of bread, ½ a bagel, one tortilla, five crackers, ½ cup rice or pasta, ¾ cup cereal
Protein foods	3–4	2 oz meat, fish, or poultry (usual serving size is about 3 oz); ½ cup dried beans; ½ cup nuts or seeds; 4 oz tofu; ½ cup cottage cheese; 2 oz hard cheese
Dairy products	4–5	1 cup low-fat or skim milk, 1 cup low-fat yogurt, 1½ cups frozen yogurt or low-fat ice cream, 1–2 oz low-fat cheese
Fruits and vegetables	5–9 (including 2 or more servings of vitamin C–rich fruits and vegetables and leafy green vegetables)	½ cup corn, green beans, or green peas; 1 medium apple; ½ banana; 10–12 grapes; ½ cup orange juice; ½ cup strawberries; 1 stalk broccoli; 1 whole tomato; ½ cup spinach

As you can see, eating all those servings from each food group leaves you very little room for things like soda, candy and sweets, or fat-filled sauces and spreads. That's where the cutting down on some foods comes in. A USDA analysis of Americans' dietary habits found that only one-fourth to one-third of people eat the recommended portions of foods in *every* food group. It's not that people aren't eating enough food, as the rising rates of overweight and obesity tell us. Instead, most people get too many of their calories from foods such as saturated fats and sweets, which pad our diets with extra calories that keep us from eating enough of the healthy foods we need. But rather than focusing too much on what you're cutting out, think about changing the balance of your diet by adding healthier foods.

How to Bring Your Diet into Balance

Most of us aren't used to thinking about our diet on a monthly, weekly, or even daily basis. We live from meal to meal. Very few people actually follow the guidelines for a balanced diet, and it's easy to see why. It would take a lot of effort to keep track of every type of food you eat, assign it to a category, and tally up the total in each category every day. Here are a few simple tricks to help bring your diet into balance:

• *Make it square.* One of the simplest ways to achieve a balanced diet is to make every meal or snack a balance of different food groups. It's what used to be called a "square meal," and it's a concept that has unfortunately dropped out of our consciousness. Following the old-fashioned square meal approach will go a long way toward making sure that your diet includes the right mix of nutrients your baby's body needs to grow. Try to make sure that all meals include a portion of food from each food group. For snacks throughout the day, try to include foods from at least two groups in each snack, and make sure you rotate through different food groups to keep your bases covered. For example: hummus on whole wheat pita, cottage cheese with carrot sticks, yogurt mixed with fruit chunks or berries, a small handful of nuts with an orange. See Chapter 9.

• *Include vegetables and fruit at every meal and snack.* The most glaring imbalance in most Americans' diets is the lack of vegetables and fruits. Most people fall far short of the goal of five servings of fruits and vegetables a day set by health authorities such as the National Cancer Institute. If you eat three meals and two snacks every day, you should include at least one serving of fruits or vegetables each time you eat. Taking this step will make a big change in the balance of your diet.

• *Change your proportions.* Studies have found that people tend to overestimate the amount of vegetables and fruit they eat in a day, while they often underestimate the amount of carbohydrates and other foods they eat. At meals, vegetables and fruits should take up a large portion of your plate. For instance, a side salad should take up half the plate, with the other half devoted to other foods. Rather than trying to ban unhealthy foods, think about changing the proportions of your diet so that healthy foods take a greater role. Start limiting the portion sizes of unhealthy foods while boosting the portions of healthy ones. For instance, if you crave sugar after a meal, reduce the amount of ice cream you typically eat at dessert while adding sliced fruit or berries as a topping. Or, instead of a large cookie for a snack, eat only half a cookie with a banana. See Chapter 9 for more healthy recipes and snack ideas.

• *Find healthy substitutes for high-fat and high-sugar foods.* Trying to radically alter your eating patterns can backfire if the changes are difficult to maintain over the months you are pregnant. In other words, it's OK to eat that favorite pastry you love or indulge in a rich meal at your favorite restaurant once in a while. But if you notice that foods that are high in saturated or trans fat and sugar are eating up a big part of your daily food intake, it's time to start making simple changes to bring more nutritious foods into your diet. Identify some simple substitutes for your indulgences that are healthier but that you can live with. For instance, use low-fat or fat-free dairy products in recipes that call for a lot of cheese, butter, or cream. Use a vegetable-based spread, such as hummus or baba ghanoush, instead of butter or cream cheese on your bagel. Replace sweets with fruit. Whole fruit—or canned or dried fruit without added sugar—can help add vitamins, minerals, and fiber to your diet while still satisfying a sweet tooth.

• *Put your indulgences to work.* What makes junk foods "bad"? In many cases, they are foods that provide us calories and things we don't need without providing any of the things we *do* need. You can put those "empty-calorie" foods to work for your health if you use them creatively as a way to add more of the healthy foods you might be tempted to skimp on. If you love desserts, dip nourishing fruit chunks in chocolate sauce or whipped topping as a way to add more produce to your diet. Or use a little creamy cheese sauce if it helps you to eat more vegetables. By working *with* your desires, rather than against them, you'll be able to make healthy changes you can live with. And adding healthier foods into the mix will help you use those "empty" foods more sparingly.

Managing Food Cravings

The strange food cravings of pregnant women are often a source of humor in popular culture. While you may not necessarily crave pickles and ice cream, most women do find that they have an inexplicable desire for foods or food combinations that they never had before, or they feel an aversion to foods they normally like. No one

How It Looks in a Day

This sample menu illustrates how to choose foods throughout the day that add up to a balanced diet.

Breakfast

1 cup granola or muesli = 2 grains
1 cup skim milk = 1 dairy
1 banana = 1 fruit

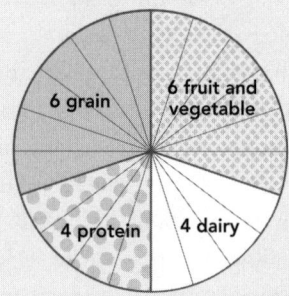

Snack

1 apple, sliced = 1 fruit
1 cup yogurt = 1 dairy

Lunch

Chicken sandwich with grilled chicken breast, 1 slice cheese, and 2 slices whole-wheat
    bread = 1 protein, 1 dairy, 2 grains
Side salad with romaine lettuce, tomatoes, and carrots = 1 vegetable

Snack

Whole Wheat Dipping Chips (see recipe in Chapter 9) = 1 grain
½ cup Sweet Roasted Garlic and White Bean Dip (see recipe in Chapter 9) = 1 protein

knows exactly why. Some pregnancy hormones might explain why some women experience unexplained food cravings and aversions during pregnancy. It's tempting to think that the cravings result from a real nutritional need—from the body "knowing" that it lacks a certain nutrient. Occasionally this might be true, but often the things that pregnant women crave don't seem to have any basis in a physical need and may even be harmful to their health if indulged too much. Cravings can make eating well more difficult by forcing you to manage a whole new set of preferences that are unfamiliar to you.

It's fine to feed your cravings as long as they fall within your goals for a healthy diet. Never allow your cravings to cause you to eat the same thing day after day—a monotonous diet can leave you lacking in important nutrients. Find compromises that satisfy your cravings in healthy ways. If you feel an aversion to certain healthy

Dinner

Tilapia Tapenade (see recipe in Chapter 9) = 2 protein and
    1 vegetable
½ cup steamed spinach = 1 vegetable
½ cup brown rice = 1 grain

Dessert

1 cup low-fat frozen yogurt = 1 dairy
½ cup strawberries = 1 fruit
Total: 6 grains, 6 fruits and vegetables, 4 dairy, and 4 proteins

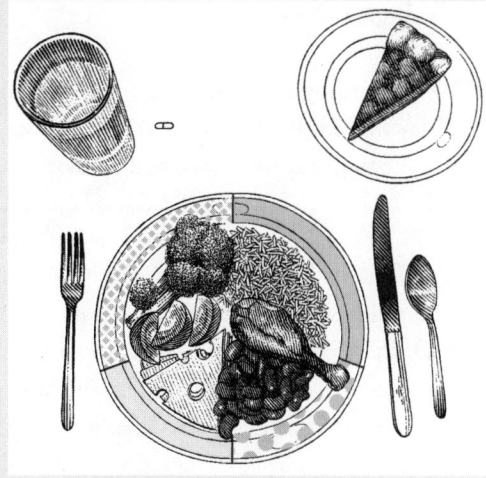

A balanced diet during pregnancy includes a variety of fruits and vegetables, grains, protein foods, and dairy, plus a daily prenatal vitamin and plenty of water. Keep added sugar and saturated and trans fats to a minimum—use small portions or add sparingly to flavor food.

foods, make the effort to find good substitutes for the nutrients you will miss. For instance, if you feel an aversion to meat, as some women do, substitute other foods rich in protein such as yogurt, milk, beans, nuts, tofu, chickpeas, or lentils, and make sure you are getting enough iron from supplements and iron-rich foods.

Occasionally, cravings can even go beyond foods. Some pregnant women find that they have unexplained desires to eat nonfood items—dirt, clay, ashes, ice, chalk, plaster, toothpaste, coffee grounds, laundry starch, and other bizarre fare— a condition called pica. Obviously, giving in to these cravings could expose you to some strange substances that may be harmful to your body and your baby. If you experience pica, don't listen to your cravings but talk to your doctor. In some studies, pica has been linked to iron deficiency, and it may be worthwhile to see your doctor in case of any underlying nutritional problems.

Nausea and Vomiting

"Morning sickness" is a bit of a misnomer, because many pregnant women find that nausea strikes any time of the day. Nausea is usually worse at the beginning of pregnancy and almost always fades by the seventeenth week of pregnancy. Until then, it's important to try to find relief from nausea and not let it interfere with your own health and nutrition.

- Avoid eating too much at a time—eating many small meals throughout the day may keep you from getting an upset stomach.
- Take time out for meals, and eat slowly.
- If smells such as coffee, fried foods, and home cooking that once smelled delicious to you now make you sick, find ways to avoid these odors in your daily routine. If cooking makes you nauseous, try instant foods or healthy takeout dishes, or have someone else do the cooking for you.
- Don't skip your meals and snacks, even if you feel like avoiding food altogether. It's important to keep nourishing your body, and keeping a little food in your stomach will help keep it from getting upset.
- Make sure you get enough sleep and rest when needed. If your nausea comes on in the morning, take your time getting out of bed. Keeping some crackers by your bed and eating a little before getting up can help.
- Greasy, spicy, or fried foods may be particularly offensive to your senses— try choosing blander foods. Avoiding fried foods will help you eat healthier as well.
- Keep drinking fluids, especially if you are vomiting. It's important to stay hydrated.

Why women's bodies react in this paradoxical way during pregnancy is a mystery, but be reassured that babies have a remarkable ability to grow properly despite your nausea. If the nausea is so severe that you are vomiting regularly or simply can't stand to eat, consult a doctor or dietitian to find ways to manage it. You should be especially concerned if you find you are eating less than you normally do or if you are not gaining as much weight as you should. If eating enough of the right foods becomes a problem, some women benefit by drinking nutritional supplement shakes, which they find easier to tolerate.

Diet and Gestational Diabetes

About 5 percent of women experience gestational diabetes, which is the development of high blood sugar and diabetes only during pregnancy. Even if you have never had problems with your blood sugar before, the dramatic changes that your metabolism undergoes during pregnancy can sometimes send your blood sugar out of balance, putting both you and your baby at risk for health problems. Fortunately, there are ways to treat gestational diabetes, especially if it's caught early, and taking special care with your diet can help you control it.

During pregnancy, the levels of hormones in your body shift. Your placenta releases hormones of its own, which can interfere with another of the body's hormones, insulin. Insulin is a signal that is responsible for telling your cells to absorb sugar from your bloodstream for energy. When insulin doesn't function properly, the sugar stays in your blood and can cause serious health complications. Normally, a pregnant woman churns out three times the normal level of insulin to counteract the hormones in her placenta. But in some cases, even this extra insulin isn't enough to keep blood sugar normal. Gestational diabetes usually shows up later in pregnancy and is usually detected by a blood test after about the twenty-fourth week of pregnancy. The diabetes generally goes away after you lose your placenta during your delivery.

Gestational diabetes does not cause your baby to develop diabetes, but it may put your child at higher risk for developing diabetes as an adult. It also does not cause serious birth defects but may result in health problems at birth and may increase the weight and size of your baby at birth, a condition that is associated with a higher risk of obesity later in life.

Women with gestational diabetes need to monitor their blood sugar levels and may require medications or insulin injections. In addition to the medical regimen outlined by your doctor, you can take special care to control your blood sugar through your diet:

- Maintain a healthy weight, and gain only the recommended amount of weight (see Chapter 7).
- Stay active by getting moderate exercise (see Chapter 8).
- Pay special attention to the carbohydrates in your diet, and limit excess sugars. Your doctor may recommend cutting back on carbohydrates to control

your blood sugar. Eating smaller portions of carbohydrates will also help you avoid overloading your blood with extra sugar all at once. Carbohydrates are an important energy source for you and your baby, so don't simply cut out carbs without discussing an eating plan with your doctor or nutritionist.

- Eat plenty of fiber, including whole-grain foods, fruits, vegetables, and legumes. Fiber can help control the levels of sugar in your blood.
- Follow a predictable eating schedule with several small meals and snacks throughout the day, including a small snack at night. This will help keep blood sugar levels steady.
- As you monitor your blood sugar levels, keep track of how they change with time of day, food consumption, and physical activity. By making note of these relationships, you can help identify the best patterns for your body.

Women who experience gestational diabetes are at a higher risk for developing diabetes after pregnancy. You should continue the healthy habits you develop even after you are pregnant to keep your metabolism healthy.

Eating Well During Pregnancy: The Bottom Line

Diet during pregnancy is not just a list of "don'ts." It's just as important to make room for healthier foods and change eating habits for the better.

- Pay special attention to getting enough calories, protein, iron, folate, and vitamin C in your diet.
- Stay hydrated by drinking water regularly, and choose beverages that add nutrients to your diet, such as skim milk and 100 percent fruit juice.
- Choose foods within each food group that maximize important nutrients, such as fiber, protein, healthy fats, vitamins, and minerals, while limiting foods that contain saturated and trans fats or too many simple carbohydrates and added sweeteners.
- Bring the food groups into balance by eating the proper proportion of each type of food every day. For most people, this means adding more fruits and vegetables as well as whole grains, protein-rich foods, and dairy products at every meal, while limiting sweets, refined carbohydrates, and high-fat foods that crowd out more nutritious choices.

5

What to Avoid
While Pregnant

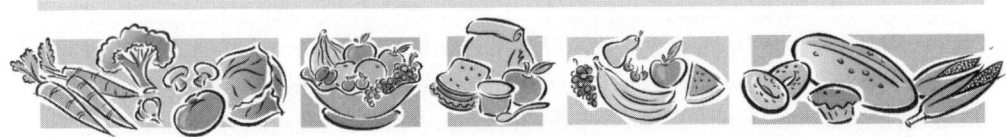

Now that we've talked about how to make positive changes in your diet during pregnancy, let's take a look at some of the "don'ts." One of the most important things you can do for your child is avoid substances that might be harmful, including those we know to harm growing fetuses. Gone are the days when pregnant women would enjoy a smoke and an afternoon cocktail and think nothing of it. We now know much more about how a mother's diet, behaviors, and environment during pregnancy can affect her baby. Birth defects and problematic pregnancies caused by smoking, drinking, and taking harmful substances are still a significant problem, but fortunately, awareness about the dangers of these habits is becoming more widespread.

However, there's a reason I saved a discussion of things to avoid until after we had talked about good nutrition. Too often these days there is undue emphasis on all the foods that pregnant women should not eat, which can leave women scared of hurting their children if they make one wrong move. And by focusing on the negatives, it's easy to lose sight of all the positive changes you can make to your diet to nourish your baby. Only a few kinds of foods or food ingredients pose a danger during pregnancy. Some of these can be a safety hazard because of toxic additives or the potential for contamination with bacteria or parasites. But with all the anecdotes, news reports, and rumors about what's bad during pregnancy, women can be left feeling as if *everything* is dangerous. Pregnant women need to be vigilant during pregnancy, but there's no reason they should be afraid to live a reasonably normal life.

It's also important to have a sense of scale. Most substances that pregnant women are told to avoid are thought to either inflict a *spectrum of harm* on a fetus, depending on the exposure, or contribute to an *increased risk* of an unwanted outcome. Alcohol is one example of a substance that is absolutely known to harm a fetus, but the level of harm is a spectrum depending on how much a mother drinks and for how long. Because it's generally not worth the pleasure of a few drinks to cause *any* potential harm to your baby, I encourage you not to drink at all during pregnancy. An example of a behavior that carries an increased risk is that of eating unpasteurized dairy products, which can raise the risk of listeriosis in pregnant women. In this chapter, I'll give you a set of safety precautions that can lower your risk of contracting this very rare illness. In this case, the possibility of harm is extremely low, but because the harm could be potentially serious and the precautions are not too drastic, it's worth following them for the months you are pregnant.

More important than worrying over a list of don'ts is cultivating an attitude of reasoned caution about the substances you eat, breathe, and expose your body to. It's unfortunate that much of what we know about which substances are off-limits during pregnancy came from trial and error. To prevent the tragedies that occur when fetuses are exposed to harmful agents, women should use caution when consuming or exposing themselves to substances that could potentially harm their babies.

Alcohol

Drinking alcohol during pregnancy can directly interfere with your baby's development. In its most extreme form, drinking alcohol during pregnancy can lead to a form of developmental impairment called fetal alcohol syndrome (FAS). FAS is a leading cause of preventable mental retardation and birth defects; children with FAS have abnormal facial features, poor growth, developmental and learning deficiencies, hyperactive behavior, poor reasoning skills, and problems with day-to-day living.

FAS is usually found in cases of very heavy drinking in mothers, and there has been much controversy over what the proper limits on drinking alcohol during pregnancy should be. What about moderate or light drinking? In fact, further research has shown that FAS is only the most severe form of alcohol's negative effects on fetal development. Every time a pregnant woman drinks, her fetus is exposed to alcohol. Alcohol has direct effects on nerve cells that interfere with their proper development. With high doses repeated over months, alcohol exposure results in severe impairments in how the brain and nervous system function. But at more moderate doses, the effects may be more subtle, including small changes in mental performance and brain function. In addition to these effects, drinking alcohol can also lead to spontaneous abortion and other pregnancy complications.

In this spectrum of harm, there is really no safe level of drinking during pregnancy. All pregnant women should avoid drinking alcohol. As we discussed in Chapter 1, damage can occur very early during an embryo's development, so you should also avoid alcohol if you may become pregnant and from the very start of pregnancy. Women who have difficulty stopping alcohol use because of addiction or other emotional problems should make every effort to seek treatment. If you are planning a pregnancy, I encourage you to stop drinking before trying to become pregnant. But it's very common for a woman to have had a few drinks before she finds out she is pregnant. If this happens, there is no reason to panic or worry that you've hurt your baby; just focus on avoiding alcohol for the rest of your pregnancy.

Smoking

Cigarette smoking by pregnant women is a primary cause of low birth weight in infants in industrialized countries such as the United States. Babies born to heavy smokers can suffer from poor growth in the womb and other health problems such as lung defects, neurological damage, and an increased risk of sudden infant death syndrome (SIDS). Because of these risks, women should make an effort to quit smoking before they become pregnant if they are planning a pregnancy, or as soon as they find out about an unexpected pregnancy. They are not only doing their babies a favor. Women who smoke live shorter lives on average and have a greater risk of dying of lung and other cancers, heart disease, stroke, and chronic lung diseases such as emphysema. Given the high price that smokers pay for their habit, giving up smoking is the single most important thing they can do for their own health.

If you smoke, helping your baby stay healthy can be a great impetus to kick a habit that may bring severe health consequences to you later in life. If you have difficulty quitting on your own, enlist family, friends, or support group, or see your doctor about setting up a treatment plan. Nicotine-replacement therapies in the form of gum, inhalers, or skin patches can help some people curb their addiction, but the nicotine still carries a risk of harming the fetus. Given that cigarette smoke contains three thousand chemicals that could potentially harm a fetus, however, nicotine replacement is at least a "lesser evil" than continuing smoking. If you feel you need to use one of these therapies to quit smoking, check with a doctor about dosage, so that you can use the lowest dose possible to minimize risks.

Secondhand smoke may also be a danger to women who are regularly exposed to cigarette smoke in their work or home. Environmental cigarette smoke is considered a carcinogen and has been shown to raise the risk of cancers in nonsmokers. A recent analysis of pregnancy outcomes and secondhand smoke exposure in three thousand women found that exposure to secondhand smoke is associated with poor fetal growth, and very high levels of exposure are associated with higher rates of fetal death and preterm birth. While you may have limited control over your environment, it's important to reduce your exposure to smoke as much as possible. This may include talking with employers about smoking policies in your workplace, setting rules about smoking in your home, or helping a smoker you live with to quit.

Caffeine

Caffeine is not a clear-cut case like alcohol. Caffeine has not been shown to cause direct damage to fetal tissues the way alcohol does, so there is some disagreement about a safe level of caffeine during pregnancy. Studies have found that excessive caffeine intake is associated with a higher risk for miscarriage and low birth weight. Too much caffeine also causes increased numbers of birth defects in laboratory animals, though it has not been linked to birth defects in humans.

The effects of moderate caffeine intake during pregnancy are not known. But even without clear evidence, we know that caffeine is a powerful stimulant that causes chemical changes in the body that could potentially affect a developing fetus.

When faced with substances such as caffeine where the evidence is not clear, pregnant women should opt for a conservative approach. It's best to cut caffeine from your diet or limit caffeine intake during pregnancy. If you do continue to drink caffeinated beverages, keep your coffee consumption to a serving or two per day—and a serving means a *small* cup of coffee or espresso drink, not a grande Starbucks coffee! Better yet, switch to drinking tea, which is much lower in caffeine. Green tea has less caffeine than black tea, making it the best caffeinated option. Decaffeinated teas and coffees have only small amounts of caffeine, and herbal teas are generally caffeine free. But beware of teas that contain added caffeine or stimulants such as ginseng or guarana—these ingredients can raise the caffeine content of the drink considerably. Choose caffeine-free sodas, or better yet, drink healthier seltzer water, skim milk, or fruit juice instead.

One of the biggest dangers of caffeine is that it's hard to know how much you're getting. The current trend of larger portion sizes of beverages means that a soda at a movie theater or restaurant can carry much more caffeine than you think. Chocolate also contains caffeine, especially dark chocolate. And many "energy" drinks contain a lot of caffeine; because their caffeine content is unknown, you should avoid these drinks in pregnancy. Brewed tea and coffee can vary widely in caffeine content, depending on how much is used and the brewing method and time. Strong gourmet coffees can have twice as much caffeine as what you might brew at home. Table 5.1 lists the caffeine content of some common foods and beverages.

If you are a caffeine addict, cutting back may not be as hard as you think. Coffee and caffeine in general are among the more common aversions that pregnant women experience. Whether this is a protective action or simply a fluke of nature, many pregnant women find that they suddenly can't stand the smell of coffee.

Recreational Drugs

It's probably no surprise that taking recreational drugs is harmful during pregnancy. Marijuana crosses the placenta and affects fetal tissues, and marijuana use has been linked to low birth weight and withdrawal symptoms—such as excessive crying and tremors—in infants. Cocaine slips through the placenta easily and can constrict blood vessels, squeezing off a fetus's oxygen supply. Opiates—heroin, methadone, and morphine—can cause addiction in the fetus and pregnancy complications. And amphetamine use can cause heart problems and other birth defects. Injecting these drugs also raises the likelihood of developing an infection such as

Table 5.1   Caffeine Content of Selected Foods and Beverages

FOOD OR BEVERAGE	CAFFEINE CONTENT
Nongourmet coffee (8 fl oz, brewed, drip method)	85 mg–135 mg
Starbucks coffee, short (8 oz)/tall (12 oz)	235 mg/335 mg
One shot (1 oz) Starbucks espresso	35 mg
Grande (16 oz) Starbucks caffe latte	70 mg
Decaffeinated coffee (8 oz brewed)	3 mg
Iced tea (8 oz)	25 mg
Black tea (8 oz)	50 mg
Green tea (8 oz)	30 mg
Coke (8 oz)	24 mg
Pepsi (8 oz)	27 mg
Mountain Dew (8 oz)	37 mg
Barq's Root Beer (8 oz)	15 mg
Hot cocoa (8 oz)	6 mg
Chocolate milk (8 oz)	5 mg
Milk chocolate (1 oz)	6 mg
M&M's, plain (¼ cup)	8 mg
Dark semisweet chocolate (1 oz)	20 mg
Chocolate-flavored syrup (1 fl oz)	4 mg

HIV. If you use illegal drugs socially, you should stop when you plan on becoming pregnant or, if that is not possible, as soon as you find out you are pregnant. If you are addicted to an illegal drug, seek help immediately, either through your health-care provider or from the organizations listed in the References. There are similar dangers in abusing over-the-counter drugs or prescription medications such as sedatives.

Medications

Many women face a difficult dilemma when deciding whether to continue to take over-the-counter and prescription medications during pregnancy. This section is intended to familiarize you with some of the issues surrounding medications in

Preferred Over-the-Counter Drugs in Pregnancy

If you need to reach for a remedy for common ailments such as headache, diarrhea, or congestion, these are the drugs thought to be safest for occasional use at the recommended dose. Some medications, such as decongestants, may cause harm if taken for extended periods of time. As with all medications, talk to your doctor first before taking them:

- **Pain reliever:** acetaminophen (Tylenol)

- **Decongestant:** pseudoephedrine hydrochloride (Sudafed)

- **Antihistamine:** chlorpheniramine (Chlor-Trimeton)

- **Antidiarrheal:** kaolin and pectin (Kaopectate)

- **Antacids:** calcium carbonate (Tums), aluminum hydroxide/magnesium hydroxide (Maalox)

- **Antigas:** simethicone (Mylanta Gas)

Avoid any multisymptom allergy or cold medicines that contain alcohol. Many of the medicines listed here are fine for occasional symptom relief but may be harmful if taken for extended periods of time. For example, constantly taking Tums can result in dangerously high calcium levels. Talk to your doctor if you need a medicine for more than a few days at a time for a chronic condition to find the safest option.

pregnancy. It is not a comprehensive discussion and should not be used to make medical decisions without the guidance of your doctor.

Some medications can cross the placenta from your bloodstream and interfere with your baby's development. Others can indirectly harm your pregnancy by affecting how your placenta can deliver nutrients or by causing your uterus to contract and trigger early labor. But other drugs either don't cross the placenta or don't have a harmful effect on a fetus. In many cases, we simply do not know for sure how a particular drug might affect a fetus, especially newer drugs. And with more and more people taking one or more prescription medications, the potential for harmful effects during pregnancy is very real. Making decisions about taking medications can be a frustrating process—your doctor may not be able to give you a simple answer, but he or she can help you weigh the benefits and risks.

In addition to prescription medications, over-the-counter drugs can also be unsafe. For example, aspirin should be avoided during pregnancy, especially during the last three months, as well as other nonsteroidal anti-inflammatory drugs (NSAIDs) such as ibuprofen (Advil, Motrin) or naproxen (Alleve). Some people mistakenly believe that anything bought without a prescription is benign, not realizing that they should consult their doctor before taking these drugs.

The FDA "grades" every medication based on what's known about its safety during pregnancy:

- *Category A.* These are drugs that have been tested for safety during pregnancy and have been found to be safe. They include supplements such as folic acid and vitamin B_6 as well as thyroid medicine in moderation, or in prescribed doses.

- *Category B.* These drugs have been used frequently during pregnancy and do not appear to cause birth defects or other problems. They include drugs such as some antibiotics, acetaminophen (Tylenol), famotidine (Pepcid), prednisone (cortisone), and insulin. Ibuprofin (Advil, Motrin), naproxen (Aleve), and some other non-steroidal anti-inflammatory drugs (NSAIDs) are considered category B *before* the third trimester but category D late in pregnancy because they can complicate labor.

- *Category C.* These are drugs that are more likely to cause problems for the mother or fetus, or drugs for which safety studies have not been finished. The majority of these drugs do not have safety studies in progress. They often come with a warning that they should be used only if the benefits of taking them outweigh the risks. They include the antifungal medication fluconazole (Diflucan), the over-the-counter decongestant pseudoephedrine (Sudafed), the antibiotic ciprofloxacin (Cipro), and some antidepressants.

- *Category D.* These drugs have clear health risks for the fetus and include alcohol, the manic depression treatment lithium, the anticonvulsant phenytoin (Dilantin), and chemotherapy drugs to treat cancer. In some cases, chemotherapy drugs are given during pregnancy if the mother's health is at stake.

- *Category X.* These drugs have been shown to cause birth defects and should *never* be taken during pregnancy. They include Accutane, a drug used to treat cystic acne; the psoriasis medications Tegison or Soriatane; and the sedative thalidomide. These medications should be halted before pregnancy if possible, or as soon as you know or suspect you are pregnant.

Many drugs in addition to the examples listed here have potential risks during pregnancy. The category system is not perfect, and the FDA is looking into changing the way it communicates risk about drugs. The surest way to learn about a drug's effects is to conduct a randomized controlled clinical trial, in which one group of people is assigned a drug and another group is given a placebo for a certain length of time. Conducting these kinds of trials in pregnant women is often unethical, given the potential risk to a fetus. So information about a drug's safety is often extrapolated from animal studies or from effects on nonpregnant women or by observing the effects of drugs in pregnant women who choose to take them once they are on the market. It's best to review all your medications, including over-the-counter drugs, with your doctor before you become pregnant, because the harmful effects of medications often happen in the first critical days and weeks of life. If you already are pregnant, check with your physician about whether it's safe to continue taking the medications. Some medications are harmful only at the beginning or end of pregnancy, so timing can be an important issue.

If an over-the-counter drug is more of a convenience than a necessity, you may want to refrain from taking it. For instance, if you are used to reaching for pain relievers, digestion aids, or cold and allergy remedies at the first sign of any symptom, you may want to use them only when you feel you really need them. But when a medication is really necessary for a medical condition, the benefit of keeping you healthy often outweighs the potential risks. For instance, if you develop an infection that must be treated with antibiotics, such as toxoplasmosis or listeriosis, you can put your baby's health (and life) at risk if you refuse or forgo treatment. Or, if you have a chronic illness that requires medications, skipping or withdrawing medicines can endanger your pregnancy if your illness is not under control. Remember that your baby's health ultimately depends on your own, and taking care of yourself is important, too.

The use of antidepressants in pregnancy has been particularly controversial. Depression affects about 10 percent of pregnant women, and the changes in hormone levels that women experience during and after pregnancy can make them particularly susceptible to mood disorders. But information about the safety of antidepressants in pregnancy is limited. Information gathered from women who have used antidepressants suggest that the newer selective serotonin reuptake inhibitors (SSRIs), such as Prozac, Paxil, and Zoloft, as well as older tricyclic medications do

Unexpected Pregnancies, Unintended Exposures

If your pregnancy is unplanned, you're not alone: nearly half of pregnancies in the United States are unintended. Without the benefit of pregnancy planning, chances are you may have exposed yourself to one or more of the substances or risk factors discussed in this chapter before you knew you were pregnant. If you are worried that you may have exposed your baby to something harmful, the important thing is not to panic or try to second-guess how this exposure may affect your pregnancy. In many cases, the risks may be negligible as long as you took steps to reduce your exposure once you discovered you were pregnant. Discuss your concerns honestly with your health-care provider, and focus on the steps you can take now to keep your baby safe and healthy.

not cause birth defects or significant health problems in babies. Many physicians feel comfortable prescribing SSRIs because there is a fairly large amount of data about their safety. However, some reports have noted withdrawal symptoms in newborns and potential toxicities associated with SSRIs. Women who are being treated for depression should consult with their doctors and weigh the potential risks of antidepressants against the significant benefits they can provide to a woman's mental health; the decision will vary according to each woman's situation.

Artificial Sweeteners

Many women should cut down on sugar during pregnancy, to keep from packing their diets with empty calories and to promote more moderate blood sugar levels and a healthier metabolism. Artificial sweeteners can seem to offer the best of both worlds: no empty calories, sweet taste. One of the advantages of artificial sweeteners is that they do not raise blood sugar levels the same way caloric sweeteners do, which can be an advantage for women with gestational diabetes or other metabolic problems. But they have often been viewed with wariness because of reports that they may harm a fetus. Artificial sweeteners, in moderation, can be a safe option, but you need to be careful which ones you choose:

• *Aspartame (Equal, NutraSweet, NutraTaste)*. Aspartame does not cross the placenta, and the FDA and the American Academy of Pediatrics Committee on Nutrition consider aspartame to be safe for pregnant women to consume, as long as the level consumed is within the accepted daily intake (ADI) set by the FDA. The ADI for aspartame is 50 milligrams per kilogram of body weight (a 125-pound woman has an ADI level of 2,800 milligrams per day). If you look at the list that follows, you'll see that that level is quite high (the equivalent of more than sixteen cans of diet soda every day!). I would recommend, as a more conservative guideline that falls in step with a healthy diet, that you limit yourself to one or two servings of aspartame-sweetened foods or beverages per day. Women who have phenyl-ketonuria, a disease in which the body's ability to metabolize the amino acid phenyl-alanine is impaired, should avoid any product containing aspartame.

Aspartame in Foods

Diet soda, 12 ounces	170 milligrams
Powdered drink, 8 ounces, mixed	100 milligrams
Gelatin dessert, 4 ounces	80 milligrams
Aspartame-sweetened fruit yogurt, 8 ounces	124 milligrams
One packet tabletop sweetener	35 milligrams

• *Saccharine (Sweet'n Low).* Out of all artificial sweeteners, saccharine is the one that poses the most potential danger to a fetus. Saccharine is a weak carcinogen, or a substance that is known to promote cancer. It is able to cross the placenta and enter a fetus's tissues. Pregnant women should avoid saccharine.

• *Sucralose (Splenda).* Sucralose is made by altering a sugar molecule so that it is many hundreds of times sweeter than sugar. Because of its altered structure, sucralose is not absorbed and metabolized in the digestive system. The scant amounts that do get into the body do not seem to cross the placenta, making sucralose a very safe choice for pregnant women who want to use artificial sweeteners.

• *Stevia and herbal sweeteners.* Stevioside or stevia is an herbal sweetener derived from the stevia plant and has been used widely in Japan, as well as in South America and China. The use of stevia as a food additive has been rejected by the FDA and by governing authorities in Europe and Canada. For now, it is sold as a dietary supplement in some specialty stores. Advocates of stevia claim it is a safe, natural, calorie-free alternative to sugar. However, there has not been enough testing performed on stevia to assess whether it is safe for general use, and there is no information about how it may affect a fetus. I would urge pregnant women to avoid stevia, as they should any herbal supplement (see Chapter 6 for more information on herbal supplements). Until more rigorous testing has been performed, there is no reason to risk your baby's health by using an untested substance.

I would recommend choosing your artificially sweetened foods wisely. Artificial sweeteners may not add anything "bad" to the diet, but they don't add anything good either. Choose those artificially sweetened foods that boost your intake of healthy nutrients—such as artificially sweetened yogurt for protein and calcium—rather than just sodas and candies.

Fish, Omega-3 Fatty Acids, and Mercury— a Double-Edged Sword?

Adding fish to your diet is a great way to boost your omega-3 fatty acids as well as protein. Several studies have also shown that taking fish oil supplements, which are high in omega-3 fatty acids, is associated with a longer pregnancy and higher birth weight. Because omega-3 fatty acids are a component of brain tissue, it has been hypothesized that the developing brain of a fetus could benefit from high levels of

"Should I Worry About Peanut Allergies?"

More and more children these days seem to develop peanut allergies, and many women have become concerned that exposing their babies to peanuts in utero or during infancy might predispose them to developing this potentially life-threatening condition. Allergies generally develop in response to a protein that is present in a food or to a substance in the environment. Some babies are at higher risk for developing allergies to proteins such as the ones in peanuts. The reason for this is unknown, but high risk is often linked to the baby's parents or parents' siblings having allergies such as hay fever, asthma, or eczema. If your baby is at high risk for food allergies because of a family history, you may want to avoid peanuts and peanut products during pregnancy and while breast-feeding. However, while certain people should be cautious, peanuts don't deserve a bad rap. They are a great source of protein, monounsaturated fats, and folate, all of which are important nutrients for a growing fetus.

these fats in a mother's diet. However, there's a serious downside to eating fish: because of human pollution, some fish now contain levels of mercury that can harm a fetus's developing nervous system. Fish that pose a particular risk are large or long-lived fish that accumulate more mercury from their environment into their bodies. Fortunately, many of the most popular fish, such as tuna and salmon, have lower levels of mercury and are safe to eat during pregnancy (see Table 5.2 for mercury content of certain fish and shellfish). However, even these safer fish should be eaten only in moderation. To be safe, the FDA recommends following these simple precautions:

- Avoid eating shark, swordfish, king mackerel, and tilefish.
- Don't consume more than two or three servings of fish per week (twelve ounces or less total).
- Choose lower-mercury fish such as shrimp, canned light tuna, salmon, pollack, and catfish. Eat only up to six ounces per week of canned or fresh albacore (white) tuna, which is higher in mercury than light tuna.
- If you are planning on eating fish caught locally, you can check advisories in your state kept by the U.S. Environmental Protection Agency at http://epa.gov/waterscience/fish/states.htm. If you can't find information about a particular type of fish, eat only up to six ounces of it (a standard dinner portion), and don't consume any other fish that week.

The FDA has been criticized by some consumer groups for being too lax in its guidelines. A nationwide survey found that 8 percent of women of childbearing age had levels of mercury in their blood above the safe limit set by the EPA, suggesting that mercury toxicity could affect a relatively small but still substantial number of babies. These guidelines may change as more is discovered about mercury levels in fish, and they can be found online at cfsan.fda.gov/~dms/admehg3.html.

Pregnant women should not cut fish out of their diets; doing so would leave out a prime source of nutrients that are important for a baby's development. If your fish consumption exceeds the recommended level in a week, there's no need for concern—simply cut back the following week. The most important thing is how your intake averages out over the weeks and months of your pregnancy. In a perfect world, consuming fish every day would be ideal for boosting your omega-3 fats. As a compromise, I suggest eating a couple of servings of low-mercury fish per week and supplementing your diet with DHA or fish oil supplements (discussed in Chapter 6) or DHA-enriched eggs.

Table 5.2   Mercury in Fish and Shellfish

The numbers here are mean mercury levels measured in different kinds of seafood.
In reality, the content may vary.

FISH	MERCURY CONTENT (PARTS PER MILLION)
High Mercury (Avoid During Pregnancy)	
Mackerel, king	0.73
Shark	0.99
Swordfish	0.97
Tilefish	1.45
Lower Mercury (Eat Two to Three Servings per Week)	
Anchovies	0.04
Catfish	0.05
Clams	ND
Cod	0.11
Haddock	0.03
Herring	0.04
Lobster (spiny)	0.09
Mackerel, Atlantic	0.05
Oysters	ND
Pollack	0.06
Salmon (canned)	ND
Salmon (fresh, frozen)	0.01
Sardines	0.02
Scallops	0.07
Shrimp	ND
Trout (freshwater)	0.03
Tuna (canned, light)	0.12
Whitefish	0.07
Other Fish and Seafood (Eat More Rarely)	
Bass (saltwater)	0.27
Carp	0.14
Halibut	0.26
Lobster (northern/American)	0.31

Table 5.2   Mercury in Fish and Shellfish *(continued)*

FISH	MERCURY CONTENT (PARTS PER MILLION)
Monkfish	0.18
Orange roughy	0.54
Snapper	0.19
Tuna (canned, albacore)	0.35
Tuna (fresh, frozen)	0.38

ND = content below the level of detection.

Source: FDA. "Mercury Levels in Commercial Fish and Shellfish." www.cfsan.fda.gov/~frf/sea-mehg.html (accessed 3/17/05).

Infections: Listeriosis and Toxoplasmosis

Changes in how the immune system functions during pregnancy can put pregnant women at a higher risk of certain infections. It may surprise you that you are more susceptible to an infection even if you feel perfectly healthy during your pregnancy. But the hormonal changes in your body during this time can leave your immune system weakened enough that it is susceptible to illnesses that others may shake off easily. Two of these—listeriosis and toxoplasmosis—are discussed in this chapter because of their potential to cause harm to a fetus or interfere with a normal pregnancy. There are steps you can take to reduce the likelihood that you will acquire either of these infections, including following special food safety precautions. While it's important to follow these precautions, you should also recognize that these illnesses are extremely rare and should not cause you undue worry or fear.

Listeriosis

Food poisoning is something that few of us get overly concerned about, but a particular kind of foodborne illness poses a special danger for pregnant women. Listeriosis is an illness caused by the bacterium *Listeria monocytogenes*. It affects about 2,500 people every year in this country, and in one of five cases is fatal. While *Listeria* can infect healthy adults and children, it rarely leads to disease. But pregnant women, newborns, and adults with weakened immune systems are particularly susceptible to listeriosis; pregnant women are twenty times more likely than other healthy adults to develop listeriosis, and they account for one-third of the cases of this illness—though that is still a very small number.

Listeriosis can affect your baby's health even if you feel few noticeable symptoms. It can take days or even weeks to show symptoms, and they may be mild. Pregnant women may feel flulike symptoms with a sudden fever, chills, muscle aches, and diarrhea or stomach discomfort. Symptoms may spread to the nervous system as headache, stiff neck, loss of balance, confusion, or even convulsions. Tell your doctor if you experience symptoms like these and believe you may have eaten a contaminated product in the past two months. A blood test can check for listeriosis, and the condition can be treated with antibiotics. But because symptoms don't always appear after infection, it's important to prevent infection by following food safety precautions.

Listeria lives in soil and water and can make its way into vegetables and into meat and dairy products. It can live in refrigerated temperatures but is killed by cooking. Pasteurization of milk products or cooking of meat products can prevent contamination with *Listeria*. However, certain processed foods such as deli meats can become contaminated after cooking and before packaging. There is no way to tell whether a food contains the bacterium—instead, the only way to ensure your food is uncontaminated is to follow safe food handling precautions, including these:

- Wash raw vegetables before eating them.
- Thoroughly cook any raw meats before eating them (avoid rare meats).
- Separate raw and cooked foods during meal preparation in order to prevent cross-contamination.
- Wash all knives, cutting boards, utensils, and kitchen countertops well.
- Use only pasteurized dairy products. Pasteurization heats foods to kill any microorganisms that live in them. Most conventional milk is pasteurized, and most dairy products are made from pasteurized milk. Cheeses that are frequently unpasteurized include Brie, Camembert, feta, blue-veined cheeses, and Mexican-style soft cheeses (*queso blanco, queso fresco, panela*). Eat these cheeses only if the package says they are made from pasteurized milk, and avoid eating them at restaurants or other places where you can't verify if they are pasteurized or not.
- Do not eat refrigerated pâté or other meat spreads (canned or otherwise shelf-stable spreads are fine).

- Do not eat refrigerated smoked seafood unless it has been cooked thoroughly. Smoked fish is often called "nova-style," "lox," "kippered," "smoked," or "jerky." Canned smoked seafood is fine to eat.
- When eating hot dogs, luncheon meats, or deli meats, first cook the meat so that it is steaming hot. Avoid letting any uncooked liquid from the packaging of those meats touch other foods, utensils, and surfaces.
- Wash your hands thoroughly after touching raw meats, deli or luncheon meats, or raw vegetables.

It takes just a little extra effort and vigilance to follow these guidelines in your own home. But when you eat out, it's much more difficult to have control over how your food is prepared. You may need to be more cautious about where you eat and the foods you choose when ordering; don't be afraid to ask about ingredients. But you shouldn't feel too scared to eat out at all. While listeriosis is a serious concern during pregnancy, the number of infections is still extremely low compared to the number of unaffected pregnancies every year in this country.

Out to Lunch

Staying away from deli meats or luncheon meats unless they have been thoroughly heated can be challenging when you're out to lunch, especially if you are used to eating sandwiches regularly. Instead of that turkey on rye, try these safer options:

- Grilled chicken or chicken salad sandwich

- Egg salad sandwich

- Cheese sandwich with vegetables

- Soup

- Salads (But avoid ordering salads topped with feta, unless you are sure it is pasteurized. Request shredded cheddar or mozzarella instead.)

Toxoplasmosis

In addition to listeriosis, an infection called *toxoplasmosis* is a concern for pregnant women. The parasite *Toxoplasma gondii* infects an estimated sixty million Americans, but most people's immune systems are able to keep the parasite from causing illness. If you are infected for the first time just before or during your pregnancy, your baby can become infected. In some cases, infection can result in eye damage or mental retardation. But if you have already been infected in the past, your baby is usually protected by the immunity you've developed. Your health-care provider should test for *Toxoplasma* infection before pregnancy or at your first prenatal visit. Symptoms of infection include fatigue, fever, and swollen lymph nodes, but sometimes there are no symptoms. If detected, infection can be treated with antibiotics.

One source of infection is cat feces. If you own a cat, there's no need to get rid of your beloved pet while you're pregnant, but you should take some precautions. If possible, stay away from the cat's litter and have someone else change it. If you must change it, use disposable gloves and wash your hands afterward. Change the litter every day, because *Toxoplasma* becomes infectious one to five days after it is shed in feces. Feed your cat commercial canned or dry food and never raw meat. Keeping cats indoors can also reduce the likelihood of an infection.

Toxoplasma can also be found in raw meat and unwashed vegetables, and in soil. To avoid exposure to contaminated objects, always wash or peel fruits and vegetables before eating them. Cook meat thoroughly, and avoid tasting it until it's completely cooked. Avoid ordering raw or undercooked meats in restaurants. You can also decrease your risk of infection by freezing meat for several days before cooking it. Always wash cutting surfaces and knives in hot, soapy water. Wash hands well after spending time outdoors gardening or touching soil.

Following the best hygiene and cleanliness you can during your pregnancy will help protect you against toxoplasmosis and listeriosis, as well as other common infections such as colds, which can be even more burdensome than usual if your body is already dealing with the profound changes of pregnancy.

Other Foodborne Illnesses

Everyone is at risk for infection when eating raw or undercooked meat, fish, and eggs. It's a good idea to lower your risk of foodborne illness during pregnancy by following safe food preparation and hygiene practices and avoiding foods such as sushi made with raw fish, very rare meats, and raw or very runny eggs.

Unpasteurized juices can be sources of infectious bacteria such as salmonella and E. coli. Most commercial juices are now pasteurized, but some fresh juices sold in health-food stores may not be; check the label if you're unsure. Raw vegetable sprouts (including alfalfa, clover, mung bean, and radish) are also major causes of food-borne illness. Avoid eating raw sprouts in salads or sandwiches and cook them thoroughly when you use them in stir-fries or other dishes.

Keeping Your Environment Healthy During Pregnancy

Many women worry about how substances in their air, food, water, home, or workplace may negatively affect their babies during pregnancy. You may start wondering about your cosmetics, hair dye, and cleaning products and how they might affect your baby. Certain kinds of paints, solvents, pesticides, and cleaners have been shown to cause birth defects or promote miscarriages during pregnancy.

You should use caution when exposing yourself to inhaled chemicals such as paints, cleaning products, and solvents. Use a mask and gloves, and keep indoor spaces well ventilated when using these products. Save indoor house painting or renovation projects for later, or have someone else do them. Be especially cautious when removing old paint—many older homes have lead paint, which can be toxic to a fetus.

Very little is known about how more common day-to-day exposure to chemicals in the environment affects fetal development. Topical products such as cosmetics and hair treatments are absorbed into the body in only trace amounts and at these low levels are unlikely to harm a fetus. Still, some women choose to limit their exposure to products like these while they are pregnant. Recent studies have found that exposure to high levels of air pollution can cause genetic changes in fetuses, and air pollution has also been linked to certain kinds of birth defects. The effects are not so severe that women should be alarmed. But the findings show how important it is that we gain a better understanding about how the pollutants in our environment affect human health and fetal development.

For now, be reassured that many of the things you are exposed to every day have also been present in countless other healthy pregnancies. Use special care to keep your environment clean and healthy during your pregnancy by avoiding prolonged exposure to known toxic substances. If you are concerned that your workplace or home environment puts you at special risk, discuss your concerns with your doctor to see if there are changes you should make. And remember that your body is your baby's environment right now—taking care of yourself is the most important thing, including getting plenty of rest, avoiding stress, and keeping yourself healthy and well nourished.

What to Avoid While Pregnant: The Bottom Line

Pregnant women should not drink alcohol, smoke, or use recreational drugs during their pregnancies. If you are addicted to these substances or have trouble quitting, get help immediately. In addition:

- Limit caffeine intake to one or two servings of caffeinated beverages a day, switch to beverages lower in caffeine such as tea, or quit altogether.
- If you use artificial sweeteners, sucralose is safest, and aspartame is also safe in moderate doses (a couple servings a day is a good guideline). Avoid products containing saccharine and herbal sweeteners.
- Talk with your doctor about any medications you are taking or intend to take during pregnancy, including over-the-counter medicines. Some drugs can harm a fetus, and you may need to find alternatives.
- You can eat fish as part of a healthy diet, but follow the guidelines to avoid mercury toxicity. You can supplement fish intake with daily DHA or fish oil supplements (see Chapter 6).
- Pregnant women need to take special food safety precautions and follow excellent hygiene to avoid listeriosis and toxoplasmosis.
- During your pregnancy, pay special attention to your environment, and reduce exposure to toxic chemicals and fumes.

6

Dietary Supplements— What's Good and What's Not

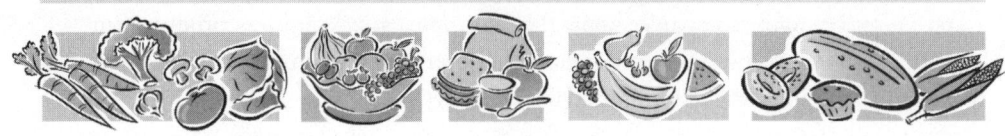

Most of your nutrient needs can and should be met by following the steps outlined in Chapter 4 for choosing healthier foods and eating a balanced diet. But you may wonder whether all the foods you eat really are enough to support the growth and development of your baby. In reality, there are sound reasons why pregnant women *should* take a little something extra beyond what their diet provides. Most physicians now recommend some kind of prenatal vitamin and mineral supplement to pregnant women to help prevent any dietary deficiencies they might have. But there are also a lot of supplements out there that are not necessary and may even be dangerous.

A dietary supplement is a product that contains a dietary ingredient that is taken out of its natural form in food and is often delivered in concentrated form. It can include vitamins and minerals, as well as herbs or other botanicals, or amino acids and other components of natural foods that have been isolated and reconstituted in another form, such as a capsule, softgel, powder, or liquid. It's important for all pregnant women to know what supplements can and can't do for them, and which ones are the ones they need.

First, I'd like to issue a cautionary note about *all* dietary supplements. Dietary supplements are regulated differently from either food or medications. The responsibility for ensuring a supplement's safety lies with the manufacturer, not an overseeing agency such as the FDA, which is responsible for taking action against any unsafe substance that reaches the market—but only after a substance has been found to be unsafe and brought to the agency's attention. With thousands of products on the market, only a very severe or widespread danger would single out one particular product. So far, the only herbal ingredient to be pulled from the market entirely has been ephedra, and then only after years of concern by health authorities. And supplements that contain the same ingredient have been found to vary widely in quality and content. This doesn't mean that all supplements are dangerous; most reputable companies know that ensuring a safe, consistent product is in their best interest. But you can't assume that everything sold on your local pharmacy's shelves has been tested for quality or safety.

Prenatal Vitamins

I have encouraged you to eat foods that are nourishing and provide a natural source of vitamins and minerals. Many foods on the market—such as breakfast cereals, beverages, and nutrition bars—are also fortified with vitamins and minerals, and these nutrients can be included in your daily tally. But there are a few critical nutrients—especially iron, calcium, and folic acid—that are difficult to get enough of through diet alone. Folic acid supplementation for women who may become pregnant and women in their first trimester of pregnancy is a key health goal in the recent federal *Dietary Guidelines for Americans* released in 2005. Most physicians recommend taking a prenatal vitamin to ensure that pregnant women are not deficient in nutrients. This is an important point, because the goal of taking a vitamin is not to "boost" the levels of any one nutrient to excess but to bring abnormally low levels of nutrients to a normal level. A reputable supplement with the right amount of vitamins and minerals can serve as a safety net in case the foods you eat fail to supply a critical nutrient that your baby needs, or if nausea and vomiting are preventing you from eating a balanced diet.

• *What's in a prenatal vitamin?* Prenatal vitamins are similar to the multivitamin formulas sold for adults—they contain a variety of vitamins and minerals that are important for health. But they are modified to meet the unique needs of pregnant women. Prenatal vitamins contain slightly higher levels of vitamins and minerals such as folic acid and iron, and they may vary slightly in other ways from general adult formulations. They come in different forms—tablets, liquid, chewable—and you can choose a form that's easiest for you to take.

• *Which one should I choose?* This is a trickier question. The dietary supplement industry is much less regulated than over-the-counter or prescription medications. It is safest to choose a supplement from a large, reputable manufacturer at a retail pharmacy, because these companies will be under higher scrutiny to provide a safe product than small companies that sell products over the Internet or in smaller stores. Choose a formula specifically designed for pregnant women, and check to see that it provides the level of vitamins and minerals that you need (see Table 6.1 for the recommended intakes for pregnant women). You can ask your doctor to recommend an over-the-counter vitamin or to prescribe one through your pharmacy. Some people may also choose not to take a multivitamin, instead preferring individual supplements of the nutrients they need most. In this case, it's important to make sure you are getting the right dose, because individual-nutrient supplements are often sold at doses above the recommended daily dose.

• *Is there a downside to taking prenatal vitamins?* As long as you are taking the proper dosage and level of vitamins and minerals, there is nothing dangerous about taking a prenatal multivitamin. However, you should never take more than the recommended dose. There is absolutely no known benefit to taking high levels of any vitamin or mineral beyond the recommended daily intake during pregnancy. You also should pay attention to the other foods you eat—if you are also eating too many foods that are fortified with high levels of vitamins and minerals, you could be consuming more of these substances than you need. Some vitamins are simply excreted as waste when you take them in excess, especially water-soluble ones like vitamin C and the B complex vitamins. But fat-soluble vitamins A, D, E, and K are stored in the liver and in fatty tissues, where they can build up over time, leading to potentially dangerous concentrations. If you were to take a multivitamin pill, eat a fortified breakfast cereal in the morning, and snack on fortified energy bars or shakes throughout the day, you could be

Table 6.1   Dietary Reference Intakes (DRIs) During Pregnancy

	NONPREGNANT ADULT WOMEN	PREGNANT WOMEN ≤ 18 YEARS OLD	PREGNANT WOMEN 19+ YEARS OLD
Calcium (mg)	1,000	1,300	1,000
Phosphorous (mg)	700	1,250	700
Magnesium (mg)	310	400	350 (360 for women 31–50 years old)
Vitamin A (mcg)	700 (2,330 IU)	750 (2,500 IU)	770 (2,560 IU)
Vitamin D (mcg)	5 (200 IU)	5 (200 IU)	5 (200 IU)
Fluoride (mg)	3	3	3
Thiamin (mg)	1.1	1.4	1.4
Riboflavin (mg)	1.1	1.4	1.4
Niacin (mg)	14	18	18
Vitamin B$_6$ (mg)	1.3	1.9	1.9
Folate (mcg)	400	600	600
Vitamin B$_{12}$ (mcg)	2.4	2.6	2.6
Pantothenic acid (mg)	5	6	6
Biotin (mcg)	30	30	30
Choline (mg)	425	450	450
Vitamin C (mg)	75	80	85
Vitamin E (mg)	15 (22.5 IU)	15 (22.5 IU)	15 (22.5) IU
Iron (mg)	18	27	27
Zinc (mg)	8	13	11
Copper (mcg)	900	1,000	1,000
Selenium (mcg)	55	60	60
Iodine (mcg)	150	220	220

Source: American Academy of Pediatrics Committee on Nutrition. Pediatric Nutrition Handbook, *5th ed.*

overloading your diet unnecessarily with these nutrients and might even approach dangerous levels of some of them.

• *Make it a habit.* If you are not used to taking a supplement every day, it can be hard to get in the habit. Try to make it part of your daily routine—for instance, keep the bottle in clear sight in the kitchen so you remember to take the pill at

Vitamin A and Birth Defects

Vitamin A is often cited as an example of the danger of taking too many vitamins and minerals as supplements. Vitamin A is one of several fat-soluble vitamins that have the ability to build up inside cells of the body. This phenomenon is a particular concern during pregnancy, because at very high doses vitamin A can cause birth defects. The highest tolerable level of intake of vitamin A for a pregnant woman has been set at 3,000 micrograms or 10,000 IU per day.

However, vitamin A is also critical for fetal cells to differentiate properly into body structures, so the need for this important vitamin is slightly higher during pregnancy. Many pregnant women have diets that are low in vitamin A, a condition that has been linked to stunted fetal growth, low birth weight, and premature delivery.

Because enough vitamin A is important but too much is dangerous, I encourage you to boost your intake by eating lots of vitamin A–rich fruits and vegetables—including leafy green vegetables, citrus fruits, winter squash, carrots, sweet potatoes, cantaloupe, and mango—rather than taking supplements (see Chapter 4 for more on vitamin A in foods). The beta-carotene in fruits and vegetables is converted to vitamin A in the body only as needed, so it is not harmful in high doses as pure vitamin A is. You can safely load up on these nutritious foods and know that the vitamin A will be there when you need it but won't when you don't. Preformed vitamin A is also found in dairy products, meat, and eggs, but you would have to eat very large quantities of these foods to approach the dangerous level found in certain supplements. Many vitamin A supplements now are made from beta-carotene rather than preformed vitamin A (also called retinol, retinyl, acetate, or palmitate). If you take a multivitamin, look for one that carries at least part of its vitamin A as beta-carotene.

breakfast or dinner. Some women find it hard to swallow large pills, especially if they are experiencing frequent bouts of nausea. Try taking the vitamin at a time of day when you are least nauseous. Chewable vitamins are available that may be easier to take. Or you can talk to your doctor about taking a combination of pills; for instance, supplements with calcium tend to be larger, so you could opt for a chewable calcium supplement along with a smaller multivitamin. Iron supplements can cause nausea in some women. You can take the iron supplement separately or not at all during the first trimester if it's very difficult to keep down, because your iron needs are less at the beginning of pregnancy.

What Supplements Can (and Can't) Do

Dietary supplements can be a critical safety net for preventing health problems that stem from deficiencies in certain nutrients. When used on large populations of people, supplements in certain vitamins and minerals have reduced rates of deficiency-related diseases, especially in poorer populations and developing countries. But it's important not to overestimate what supplements can do. Sometimes it's hard to believe that the foods you eat can really provide nearly all the nutrients your baby needs to grow and develop. Advertisers can capitalize on this doubt by convincing women that there is some other product they need in order to have the healthiest, smartest babies they can. But supplements can't take the place of eating a healthy diet. For instance, fruits and vegetables contain hundreds of chemicals in addition to vitamins and minerals that are probably important for your health. You can't "boost" your baby's health by taking more of a particular nutrient than recommended. Supplements are designed for preventing potential deficiencies; they will not benefit health when consumed at a higher level than the body needs, and some may cause serious health problems in large doses.

Your health and the health of your baby will benefit from making better dietary choices and seeking your vitamins and minerals in healthful foods rather than pills. But be realistic about your diet when deciding whether or not to take additional supplements. If you doubt your ability to cover all the bases through food alone, a supplement is a good way to ward off any potential deficiencies.

Fish Oil/DHA Supplements

There has been a lot of interest recently in fish oil supplements for pregnant women. Fish oil contains high levels of omega-3 fatty acids, especially a type called DHA (docosahexaenoic acid). These fats have graced headlines frequently in the past few years for their potential to alleviate conditions as diverse as heart disease and depression. Omega-3 fatty acids are one of the essential fatty acids, which cannot be produced within our bodies and must be found in food. They have several potential benefits to everyone, not just pregnant women: they have been shown to reduce the incidence of heart attacks and strokes; they lower the level of bad (LDL) cholesterol in your blood; they lower the amount of triglycerides in your blood.

There is no definitive answer yet as to whether women should take extra DHA during pregnancy. But there are a couple of reasons why it's probably a good idea to do so. For one, omega-3 fatty acids are a natural and healthful part of the diet and are often lacking in typical American diets. Americans consume few omega-3 fatty acids, despite the fact that this type of fat has been linked to decreased risk of heart disease and other diseases. Second, fatty acids such as DHA help form the structure of cells in the body, especially in the brain, and are needed for proper fetal development. If DHA is an important ingredient in building a healthy brain, it makes sense that pregnant women can benefit their children's development by ensuring that there is plenty of DHA in their diet. The type of fats that are available to your fetus varies with your own diet—without enough healthy fats, your baby may lack some of the necessary building blocks to form a healthy brain and body. So far, there is no evidence that consuming more of these fats during pregnancy equals smarter babies, and the actual effects are probably far more subtle. But because DHA is an unsaturated fat with known health benefits to both adults and children, adding DHA to your diet is a good step to take for your baby's health.

Research has also shown that higher consumption of fatty acids such as DHA from fish or fish oils might help prevent preterm delivery and prolong pregnancy. This theory was based on the relatively high birth weight of babies born to women living in the Faroe Islands and Scandinavian countries, who consume a lot of fish. One trial that supplemented pregnant women's diets with either fish oil, olive oil, or no treatment found that pregnancies in the fish oil group lasted an average of four days longer than those in the olive oil group, and the infants were about 100 grams heavier. Another study supplemented women's diets with eggs enriched with DHA versus regular eggs and found that pregnancies lasted an average of six days longer with higher DHA. While there is no reason to try to prolong a normal pregnancy, preterm delivery is a major cause of complications and health problems in newborns, so fish oil may be especially helpful to women with a history of delivering babies prematurely or with complications that put their babies at risk for prematurity.

The most active omega-3 fatty acids, DHA and EPA (eicosapentaenoic acid), can be found in various marine foods, including fish, seafood, seaweed, and algae. Another less active type, alpha-linolenic acid (ALA), is found in flaxseeds, canola oil, walnuts, and omega-3-enriched eggs. Fish, one of the richest dietary sources of DHA, now carry potentially harmful levels of mercury for a growing fetus. For guidelines on the safety of fish, see Chapter 5. Fish may also contain traces of other environmental toxins and pesticides, an unfortunate by-product of human pollution. While there is no reason to ban fish from your diet, it's not safe to eat fish every day. Instead, you can eat fish a couple of times a week and supplement your diet with other food sources of omega-3 fats or fish oil or DHA supplements.

Are fish oil pills safer? Like all dietary supplements, fish oil pills are only loosely regulated and their quality may vary widely. But there have been a few studies that suggest fish oil pills are generally safe. A Harvard group measured the mercury levels of five fish oil supplements and found that there were only negligible amounts of mercury in all of them, and the levels of organochlorines and polychlorinated biphenyls (PCBs)—two environmental toxins sometimes found in fish—were below the detectable limit. Another study by ConsumerLab.com found no detectable levels of mercury in twenty different types of fish oil pills. And a Consumer Reports analysis of sixteen fish oil supplements found that they did not contain significant amounts of mercury, PCBs, or dioxins. Fish oil may affect how well your blood clots, and people should avoid them if they are taking anticoagulants (anticlotting medications), have had a stroke, or are preparing for surgery. Because of their effect on clotting, it's wise to stop taking them a couple of weeks before your due date.

Fish oil pills can sometimes leave you with unpleasantly fishy breath—if so, try storing them in the freezer and taking them before you go to bed or with a large meal. There are now DHA supplements that come from nonfish sources such as algae, which may be more tolerable and are free of any toxins that may be found in fish. As with any other kind of supplement, don't overdo it. Because the research on the benefits of DHA is still unclear, the best daily dosage is unknown. Many studies have used doses from 100 to 500 milligrams of DHA, but the actual content of different pills varies. Follow the recommended dose (usually one or two softgels a day), and check with your doctor if you are unsure.

Herbal Supplements

Herbal medicines have gone mainstream in recent years. Not only do herbal supplements garner a large share of shelf space in stores these days, but herbs are also added to regular multivitamins—and even to energy bars, beverages, and snack foods. There are many herbal remedies for pregnant women that are passed on anecdotally through books, websites, and even health-care practitioners. Often these remedies are recommended early in pregnancy to ease symptoms such as nausea, toward the end of pregnancy to stimulate or slow labor, or during labor as pain relief. Many women struggle with discomforts during pregnancy but think their complaints may be dismissed by their doctors as not "serious" symptoms. Without a better way to manage symptoms, women sometimes turn to self-medicating with herbs.

No one knows how many pregnant women use herbal medications during their pregnancy. In a survey given to women late in their pregnancy at Brigham and Women's Hospital in Boston, only about 7 percent of the women reported using an herbal medication, suggesting that pregnant women may be more cautious than the general population in using these therapies. But nearly half of those who used herbs were doing so under the advice of their health-care practitioner. Most major physicians' organizations in the United States caution against taking any herbal remedies during pregnancy. But a survey of nurse-midwives in North Carolina found that 73 percent recommended herbal medications to their patients. Obviously there is a lot of disagreement even among health practitioners about whether herbs should be used.

What's so harmful about herbal medications? Herbal supplements are a huge question mark in health today. While many herbal additives are advertised as "natural" and therefore less harmful, any herb has the potential to be toxic, and the vast majority of herbal supplements has not been studied to the same extent as medications approved by the FDA. Another question mark with these products is dosage—there is currently no way to know how much of an herbal substance any product contains, what dose is considered effective, or how much is too much.

If the safety of herbal products is unclear for the general population, their safety for pregnant women and their fetuses is even more unknown. The tiny size of a fetus relative to an adult serves to magnify any biological effects of drugs and other substances that can travel across the placenta. Even substances that have been used by adults for many years with few side effects could potentially harm a developing fetus. An herb may also affect your body in a way that has consequences for your pregnancy. For example, garlic, feverfew, ginger, ginkgo, and ginseng have all been reported to affect blood circulation, suggesting they may exacerbate bleeding during labor. Certain herbs have also been known to cause uterine contractions if taken in concentrated doses, which could provoke a miscarriage or premature labor—some of these, such as blue cohosh, have been used traditionally to induce labor at the end of pregnancy.

It's not just the herbs themselves that may be harmful. A recent study published in the *Journal of the American Medical Association* tested several ayurvedic herbal remedies from India that were sold in stores in Boston and found that one in five of them contained potentially harmful levels of at least one of three heavy metals—lead, mercury, and arsenic. These levels are above the safety limits set for adults, and they would pose even more danger to a fetus.

Are any herbs safe? Herbs or foods that you use to flavor your meals are fine; it's only when they are put into concentrated doses in pills that they are worrisome. Similarly, herbal teas are also fine to drink, because they are weaker forms of the herb, and relatively little of the plant makes its way into your body. But it's best to limit yourself to two eight-ounce servings a day. Large amounts of certain herbal teas such as peppermint and red raspberry leaf have been linked to uterine contractions that may increase the risk of miscarriage or preterm labor. Herbal teas are also sometimes "supplemented" with concentrated herbs to promote an effect in the body. Stick with conventional teas that don't have additives. Avoid any vitamins or foods that have herbs added to them (often the product will claim to ease stress, aid memory, lift mood, or perform some other function beyond the product's intended purpose).

In the past several years, an increasing number of clinical trials have been launched to help determine the efficacy and safety of herbal medications. But relatively few of these will address safety during pregnancy. Definitive answers will take time, and in the meantime I urge you to be cautious. If your health-care practitioner does recommend an herbal remedy, be skeptical and make sure you discuss the potential risks before you take the advice.

Other Nutritional Supplements

In addition to multivitamins, some companies sell nutritional supplements such as milkshakes designed specifically for pregnant women. There is absolutely no need to use these products if you are eating a balanced diet and including lots of nutrient-rich foods such as the ones I discussed in Chapter 4. In fact, I worry that women who use these products see them as a shortcut to a healthy diet, which they are not. Drinking a milkshake, even one fortified with protein, vitamins, and minerals, can't compare to all the benefits we get from eating natural foods such as fruits, vegetables, whole grains, legumes, lean meats, low-fat dairy products, and healthy unsaturated fats. With just a little effort, you can nearly always find a snack that is quick, inexpensive, and nutritious, rather than reaching for a shake.

Probiotics in Pregnancy

Probiotics are foods or food supplements that contain cultures of live bacteria that are beneficial to health. Unlike bacteria that cause infections and disease, the harmless bacteria living in our digestive system are actually necessary for our health and digestive function. The goal of probiotics is to deliver extra supplies of good bacteria that can set up camp in the digestive system to help improve digestion, bolster the immune system, and keep harmful bacteria out. The simplest probiotic food is plain old yogurt, which has been recognized to have health benefits for centuries. A growing body of research has looked at the potential of beneficial bacteria to prevent infections and other gastrointestinal disturbances, help the immune system protect the digestive tract, and prevent allergic conditions.

Many studies have examined the benefit of giving probiotics in infants, but there has also been some interest in their use at the final stages in pregnancy. When a baby is born vaginally, he acquires bacteria from his mother that then begins to settle into his digestive tract. Exposing babies to the right kinds of bacteria helps establish good digestive health, and some believe it may help prime the immune system and prevent allergic disease. But this hypothesis is far from proved. In one clinical trial researchers gave supplements of the beneficial bacterium *Lactobacillus GG* to pregnant women who had a family history of allergic disease. The babies born to the women on probiotics had nearly half the incidence of the allergic skin condition eczema as women given a placebo. However, the trial was a relatively small one, so more research is needed to determine whether probiotics in pregnancy can make a difference.

Unlike herbal supplements, probiotics are known to be safe because they are supplying bacteria that grow naturally in the human digestive system. While probiotic foods are widely used in Europe and other regions, in the United States very few of the commercial brands of yogurt contain enough live active cultures to function as effective probiotics. There are several kinds of probiotic supplements, usually in the form of pills or capsules. Like other supplements, these can vary widely in quality and content. A couple of brands now guarantee to deliver an effective dose of good bacteria—usually on the order of a billion bacterial cells—but other pills may simply get chewed up in digestion, keeping the bacteria from reaching the intestines where they can attach and live. Eating yogurt, especially brands that advertise a high level of live active cultures, has the benefit of boosting your protein and calcium while potentially helping to bring good bacteria into your body.

Some health-care providers do recommend nutritional supplements in exceptional cases. For instance, if you are plagued with severe food aversions or nausea and are having difficulty meeting your calorie and nutrient needs through conventional foods, drinking a shake can be a good way to add some nourishment that is convenient and easy to tolerate. Or if you have trouble swallowing pills or remembering to take vitamins every day, your health-care provider may recommend a fortified food or shake as an alternative.

If you were taking any other kind of dietary supplement before pregnancy, check with your doctor to see if you should discontinue its use while you are pregnant. Pregnant women should not take special diet foods or supplements designed for athletes, such as creatine. All you need to stay healthy should be covered by eating nourishing foods and taking a prenatal vitamin or similar supplement. Don't reach for pills or powders over real foods, and take a cautious approach about the products you consume.

Supplements in Pregnancy: The Bottom Line

Most pregnant women need a little extra help to get important nutrients such as folic acid, iron, and calcium during pregnancy. Taking a prenatal multivitamin every day will help to boost the levels of these important nutrients in your diet and prevent potential deficiencies of other vitamins and minerals. When selecting and taking a supplement, remember the following:

- Choose a reputable supplement under the advice of your health-care practitioner, and never take extra doses.
- Don't use your multivitamin as an excuse not to fill your diet with healthy, nutrient-rich foods—pills are no substitute for the real thing.
- A daily fish oil pill or DHA supplement can help boost the healthy fats in your diet and may even have health benefits for your pregnancy and your baby.
- Be wary of herbal supplements, which have not been tested for safety. Limit your herbs to the ones you put in your food and conventional herbal teas in moderation.
- Nutritional supplements, such as bars and shakes, can't replace a healthy diet and are not necessary for most pregnant women unless recommended by a doctor or nutritionist.

7

Why Weight Matters

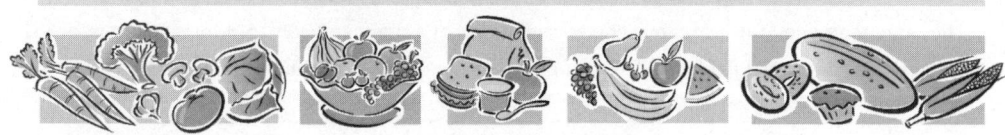

A woman's increasing weight and size are the most noticeable signs of pregnancy. It's the best indication of "how far along" she is and is her most measurable indicator of how her baby is growing. But weight is much more than just an outward change. It is an important indicator of all the internal metabolic changes a woman's body experiences, as well as of the growth of her baby. How much weight you gain during pregnancy can have a big impact on your baby's health.

Even though a healthy weight gain is one of the most important aspects of pregnancy, a large survey of women in the United States found that 27 percent received no medical advice about weight gain in pregnancy—and among those who did get advice, 14 percent were told to gain less than recommended, and 22 percent were told to gain more than recommended. Overweight women were told more frequently to gain too much weight, while African-American women, who as a group are at a greater risk of delivering babies with a low birth weight, were more likely to be told to gain too little. A more recent study of women in the San Francisco Bay area found that overweight women were more likely to set their target gain too high, and underweight women were more likely set their target gain too low—one-third received no guidance from their doctors on weight gain.

On top of this poor medical advice, add all the confusing messages about weight in our culture. Even as TV, movies, and other media regularly present nearly impossible standards of thinness for women, we are in the midst of an epidemic of over-

Where Does the Weight Go?

It's a misconception that the majority of your weight gain comes from your baby or that most of it is just extra fat. As you can see from the following table, the baby accounts for only a little more than one-fourth of the average weight gain of a pregnant woman. More weight is taken up by the added fluids needed to supply the baby with blood and nutrients.

LOCATION	WEIGHT IN POUNDS	PERCENTAGE TOTAL WEIGHT GAIN
Breasts	1	4
Placenta	1.4	5
Fluid/blood volume	8.3	30
Baby	7.5	27
Uterus	2.1	8
Other changes	7.2	26
Average total weight gain	27.5	100

Adapted from BWH Department of Nutrition patient education material.

As you can see, much of the additional weight comes from the placenta, the blood, the uterus (which expands to fit the baby), as well as additional fat tissue that holds energy stores. All of these changes are involved in delivering nutrients to the baby and creating a good environment for growth. So the weight you gain is not just excess padding—it's the entire infrastructure your body must create to help your baby grow and develop.

weight that is threatening to become one of the most widespread health problems worldwide. These days, there is increasing awareness about how excessive weight gain can cause serious health problems in children and adults and poses potentially enormous consequences for public health worldwide. All of this can make the prospect of weight gain in pregnancy all the more confusing.

Pregnancy is one of those rare occasions in adult life when it's good to gain weight and unhealthy not to. A woman must gain weight in order to have a healthy pregnancy. Too little weight gain can end up inhibiting a baby's growth in the womb and causing serious health consequences. At the same time, gaining too much weight also carries health risks for both mother and infant. In fact, improper weight gain—and its resulting effects on the growing fetus—is one of the key factors that can "program" a baby to be more susceptible to chronic disease in later life, as we discussed in Chapter 3.

Your body follows a well-defined program in pregnancy; in many ways, it "knows" what to do and will gain weight naturally. But because your weight is also influenced by your eating patterns and level of activity, you can learn to notice whether your weight gain is progressing normally and make changes if needed.

A Mother's Weight Gain Influences Her Baby's Health

Even though the baby's growth accounts for only a minority of the weight gained during pregnancy (see sidebar), there is a clear connection between the weight a mother gains and the birth weight of her infant. Birth weight is often simply an indicator of how long a pregnancy lasted (premature babies are smaller), but if a baby is small or large for the length of the pregnancy, it may be a sign of growth irregularities, which are associated with health problems in infancy and adulthood. Women who gain too little weight have a higher chance of giving birth to a smaller-than-normal baby, while women who gain too much weight have a higher chance of giving birth to a larger-than-normal baby. But somewhat paradoxically, too much weight gain and too little weight gain both can cause similar metabolic problems in a child, including a higher risk of diabetes and obesity later in life. You can think of the weight a mother gains during pregnancy as a spectrum, with the potential for health problems rising at either end. Women who are undernourished as well as those who are obese have higher rates of premature delivery, which can bring multiple health problems for babies who aren't yet fully prepared for life outside the womb.

Your Target Weight Gain

In 1990, the Institute of Medicine issued guidelines for weight gain during pregnancy based on collected evidence. The "right" amount is not a single number—it varies for each woman based on how much she weighs at the onset of pregnancy. The guidelines for weight gain are based on body mass index, a ratio of height to weight. Find your BMI by referring to Table 7.1. A normal-weight woman who has a BMI of about 20 to 26 should gain around twenty-five pounds during pregnancy. As you can see from Table 7.2, women who have a lower BMI should gain more weight during pregnancy than women with a higher BMI.

You should view these numbers as general targets. Assigning ideal numbers can be unrealistic, because women's bodies naturally vary in the changes they undergo while pregnant. A few decades ago, health authorities cautioned women to gain less weight in pregnancy, which undoubtedly led to some unhealthy behaviors as women tried to curb their weight gain through dieting or taking diuretics. The purpose of the guidelines is not to force you to compromise your health to achieve an ideal weight. Setting some targets can help you gauge whether you are nutritionally healthy during your pregnancy and make adjustments to eating habits if needed.

As mentioned earlier in this book, you can also think about the weight you gain as additional energy you take into your body. The extra energy needed for a pregnancy averages out to about 300 calories per day for a normal-weight woman. These are some examples of foods that provide 300 calories:

- Three bananas
- One ounce of low-fat cottage cheese and one ounce of dry-roasted nuts
- One cup of beans
- Two eggs scrambled with cheese
- One large bagel
- 1½ cups Caesar salad
- 1½ cups whole wheat pasta with ½ cup tomato sauce

A woman who is overweight already has some extra energy in store and may not need to consume this many extra calories beyond what she normally eats, while a woman who is underweight may need to increase her food intake a little more.

Table 7.1 Prepregnancy Body Mass Index

BMI (KG/M²) Height	19	20	21	22	23	24	25	26	27	28	29	30	35	40
	Weight (Pounds)													
4'10"	91	96	100	105	110	115	119	124	129	134	138	143	167	191
4'11"	94	99	104	109	114	119	124	128	133	138	143	148	173	198
5'0"	97	102	107	112	118	123	128	133	138	143	148	153	179	204
5'1"	100	106	111	116	122	127	132	137	143	148	153	158	185	211
5'2"	104	109	115	120	126	131	136	142	147	153	158	164	191	218
5'3"	107	113	118	124	130	135	141	146	152	158	163	169	197	225
5'4"	110	116	122	128	134	140	145	151	157	163	169	174	204	232
5'5"	114	120	126	132	138	144	150	156	162	168	174	180	210	240
5'6"	118	124	130	136	142	148	155	161	167	173	179	186	216	247
5'7"	121	127	134	140	146	153	159	166	172	178	185	191	223	255
5'8"	125	131	138	144	151	158	164	171	177	184	190	197	230	262
5'9"	128	135	142	149	155	162	169	176	182	189	196	203	236	270
5'10"	132	139	146	153	160	167	174	181	188	195	202	207	243	278
5'11"	136	143	150	157	165	172	179	186	193	200	208	215	250	286
6'0"	140	147	154	162	169	177	184	191	199	206	213	221	258	294
6'1"	144	151	159	166	174	182	189	197	204	212	219	227	265	302
6'2"	148	155	163	171	179	186	194	202	210	218	225	233	272	311
6'3"	152	160	168	176	184	192	200	208	216	224	232	240	279	319
6'4"	156	164	172	180	189	197	205	213	221	230	238	246	287	328
	NORMAL WEIGHT						OVERWEIGHT					OBESE		

Table 7.2   Recommended Weight Gain Based on Prepregnancy BMI

BMI BEFORE PREGNANCY	RECOMMENDED WEIGHT GAIN DURING PREGNANCY
<19.8 (underweight)	28–40 lbs.
19.8–26.0 (normal weight)	25–35 lbs.
>26.0–29.0 (overweight)	15–25 lbs.
>29.0 (obese)	At least 15 lbs.

The Timing of Weight Gain

The pace of weight gain varies for different people. You should expect to gain only a small amount of weight in the first trimester and then gradually begin to gain more rapidly in the second and third trimesters. Your actual weight gain will vary according to how much you weighed when you became pregnant, but these are average rates:

- *First trimester:* one pound per month
- *Second and third trimesters:* one pound per week, or three to four pounds per month

Again, these are general guidelines, not absolutes. Try to weigh yourself weekly on a scale to track your progress. Don't expect to gain the same amount of weight each week, but see how the weight gain averages over a month. Some studies have linked pregnancy complications or infant birth weight to weight gain specifically in certain trimesters, but so far no one part of pregnancy appears to be most critical. It's more important that you gain weight slowly and steadily, and that the pace of weight gain increases after the first months. Anything more sudden—no longer gaining weight or gaining several pounds rapidly—could be a sign that something is wrong and should be discussed with your doctor.

Steady weight gain may not always translate into steady eating patterns throughout pregnancy. During the first trimester, many women experience nausea and may need to make a little extra effort to eat enough. The second trimester is often the time when women can truly eat more than usual, especially as the baby's growth picks up. During the third trimester, eating can again become a chore as the growing baby pushes against your internal organs, including the stomach. Small, fre-

Multiples and Weight Gain

Twins and multiples add more weight than a singleton pregnancy, but the differences are more modest than you might think. Women carrying twins should aim for an average weight gain of thirty-five to forty-five pounds total. They should be steadily gaining a little more weight than average—about four to six pounds in the first trimester, followed by about one and a half pounds per week in the second and third trimesters. Another way to think about this is that women pregnant with twins should be taking in about 150 calories more per day than a woman carrying a single fetus—or 450 calories more than her intake before pregnancy. There is less known about triplets or beyond, but evidence so far suggests that fifty pounds total weight gain, or one and a half pounds per week through the entire pregnancy, is a healthy weight gain for triplets. It's good to start gaining weight early in pregnancy, because pregnancies with multiples are often shorter because the babies are born prematurely. Because multiple fetuses share resources and space, the additional weight that a woman puts on is increasingly due to the weight of the fetuses themselves rather than changes in her body.

quent meals and snacks in this time are the best way to fit food in while also preventing heartburn that the internal squeezing can cause.

Should You Limit Excessive Weight Gain?

Over the past few decades, American women have been gaining more weight on average during pregnancy. Some nutritionists worry that this trend of excessive weight gain is partly to blame for the rise in overweight and obesity in the United States. While weight gain is a fact of pregnancy, it's also important for women not to overestimate the amount of weight they need to put on, because too much weight gain isn't good for them or their babies. But pregnancy is not a time to diet or cut back on calories, which could compromise the nutrition you provide your baby.

Don't worry if your weight gain is a few pounds off the targets. Every woman's body is different, and you don't want to interfere with the natural unfolding of your body's changes as it supports the growth of a baby. But women who gain fifty pounds or more in their pregnancies can have real difficulties losing the extra weight after pregnancy. If your weight gain becomes excessive, see your doctor or nutritionist about whether your eating habits or activity level need to be adjusted. You may be overestimating the amount of additional food you need to eat in pregnancy. In Chapter 4 I explained why the idea that pregnant women are "eating for two" can be misleading, because it's more important to improve the quality of your diet than to increase the quantity of food you eat. The added calories needed during pregnancy—about 300 extra calories a day—isn't that much and may be even less for someone who tends to overeat. You should *never* diet or skip meals if you are gaining too much weight during pregnancy, but you can follow these tips to cut back on excess calories while still keeping your diet rich in nutrients:

- Plan to eat three small meals, with healthy snacks between meals. Never skip a meal or snack in order to cut calories; eating regularly is better for keeping your blood sugar levels even and preventing you from overeating to compensate for the hunger if you go without food for too long.
- Keep portion sizes of foods reasonable, and don't finish overlarge portions at restaurants.
- Eat slowly, and give yourself time to digest food. Always start with a small serving of food and wait a few minutes after you've finished to decide if you need seconds.
- Cut back on foods with added sugars, refined flour, and fats. These "energy-dense" foods pack a lot of calories into a small amount of space. You don't have to cut these foods out entirely, but eat only very small portions (for example, half of the typical cookie or pastry sold at bakeries is plenty).
- Fill up on fruits and vegetables, which contain lots of water and fiber that keep you full with fewer calories (and provide lots of vitamins and minerals in the meantime). Keep them handy as snacks to prevent yourself from reaching for junk foods.
- Avoid sweetened beverages or overlarge portions of other beverages such as juice. Use low-fat or fat-free milk and other dairy products.

Some women start to avoid physical activity when they're pregnant, which can contribute to unhealthy weight gain. With some care to avoid dangerous activities, pregnant women can still enjoy an active lifestyle for the majority of their pregnancy. See Chapter 8 for information about physical activity and exercise.

Being Overweight in Pregnancy

In the United States, more than half of women are considered overweight or obese based on the current definitions developed by the Centers for Disease Control. Many of those women, especially those in the lower ranges of the overweight category, might not even consider themselves to be overweight. It's important to realize that the CDC categories don't capture all the individual differences among women of the same BMI. They are not meant to be a judgment on physical appearance. Instead, the categories are meant to reflect what's known about how weight affects health and disease; women who fall into the overweight or obese categories are at higher risk for health problems and chronic disease.

In Chapter 1 I explained why reaching a healthy weight before pregnancy can help prevent pregnancy-related health problems and offset some of the risks associated with weighing too much. But losing weight and maintaining weight loss well before pregnancy is an ideal situation that not every woman can accomplish. If you are above the healthy weight range while you are pregnant, you can still have a normal, healthy pregnancy, but it's good to be aware of some of the risks that overweight and obese women face.

Women who are even moderately overweight are more likely to have problems with their metabolism, which includes all the body's systems for taking in energy from food and using that energy to power the functions of the body. Metabolic health problems include gestational diabetes and pregnancy-induced high blood pressure. Overweight and obesity also carry higher risks of miscarriage, pregnancy complications, infant mortality, delivery problems, prematurity, cesarean section, and urinary problems.

Overweight and obese women should avoid diets that put stress on their metabolism. Eating a lot of sugars and refined carbohydrates such as white flour can cause insulin and blood sugar to swing quickly and dramatically. Over time, the tissues of the body lose their sensitivity to insulin, making it difficult to clear sugar from the bloodstream and into the body. Blood sugar levels remain perpetually high, a condition that can lead to diabetes. Women who are overweight can help offset some of the metabolic complications of pregnancy by avoiding refined grains and excessive added sugars and emphasizing carbohydrates from whole grains, fruits and vegetables, legumes, and low-fat dairy products. Moderate exercise can also help to normalize metabolic health problems.

The amount of weight that obese women should gain in pregnancy is controversial. The current recommendations by the Institute of Medicine suggest that even women who are obese should gain a small amount of weight in pregnancy—fifteen pounds or more. However, a study from 1996 found that there are diminishing returns in maternal weight gain—each pound that women gain while pregnant raises the average birth weight of their infants, but this effect tapers off when overweight and obese women gain weight. In other words, at the higher end of the weight range, the extra weight women gain is increasingly adding fat to their bodies rather than helping their babies grow. The extra weight may also increase their risk of developing complications such as high blood sugar during pregnancy, also called gestational diabetes. Gaining less weight can help prevent some of the complications of pregnancy that come with obesity and can keep women from adding on extra weight that will be difficult to shed after pregnancy. More research needs to be done to figure out whether less is more for obese women, but for now, expect to gain a conservative amount of weight and focus on eating well, staying active, and not overeating.

How Can You Improve Poor Weight Gain?

Some women find it difficult to gain enough weight, especially if they are overcome with nausea and food aversions that interfere with eating a normal diet. It helps to identify foods you like and can easily tolerate and make those foods available rather than forcing yourself to eat things you don't like. Chapter 4 lists some additional tips for dealing with nausea. Be reassured that nausea is a common phenomenon during pregnancy, and babies seem to be able to grow normally in spite of it. But if you are vomiting frequently, seek advice from your doctor on how to eat enough and control the vomiting. Poor weight gain can also be a sign of stress or emotional problems such as depression, and these conditions are also important to address.

Weight gain is an outward sign that your body is providing good nourishment and encouraging your baby's growth. Think about boosting your weight gain with nutrient-rich foods that will nourish your baby, rather than eating high-calorie but unhealthy foods just to put on pounds. Some women may follow a balanced diet, eat a little more than they used to, choose healthy foods, exercise moderately, and get plenty of rest but just don't gain weight as quickly. In this case, your weight gain may be a sign of the natural variability of human bodies, and you don't need to worry over it or try to force yourself to gain more.

Is Losing Weight in Pregnancy Ever OK?

Weight loss during pregnancy can be a sign of an inadequate diet, either because the mother is not able to eat enough or because of severe nausea and vomiting or other illness. Some women may lose a little weight at the beginning of pregnancy if they begin to adopt better dietary habits and eat healthier foods, especially if they were overweight or obese to begin with. This is the body's natural response to a diet that is lower in empty calories from sweets and junk food but is actually more nourishing. However, this weight loss should soon even out, and weight should begin to rise once the pregnancy progresses. You should never intentionally lose weight or follow a weight-loss diet while you are pregnant. Gaining weight in pregnancy is not the same as getting fat. If you begin to experience weight loss beyond the first couple of months of pregnancy, talk to your doctor or nutritionist to make sure your diet is adequate.

Weight Gain in Pregnancy: The Bottom Line

Gaining the right amount of weight during pregnancy can help keep you healthy, keep your pregnancy problem free, and ensure that your baby grows properly and avoids undue risks of health problems at birth and into adulthood.

- How much weight you gain depends on how much you weigh at the outset. Though individual weight gain varies, normal-weight women should gain about twenty-five to thirty-five pounds, overweight and obese women should gain about fifteen to twenty pounds, and underweight women should gain up to forty pounds.
- The timing of weight gain is slow and steady—just a few pounds total in the first trimester, followed by around a pound a week in the last two trimesters.
- You should try to modify your weight gain only within the reasonable limits of a nourishing, balanced diet. Never try to diet or exercise excessively; instead, monitor your weight gain, focus on eating better-quality foods, and make small adjustments in your food intake and activity level if necessary.
- See your doctor if you are having difficulty gaining weight or are gaining too quickly. Overweight and obese women should also talk to their doctor about dietary changes to help them avoid metabolic problems such as gestational diabetes.

8

How to Stay Active, Safely

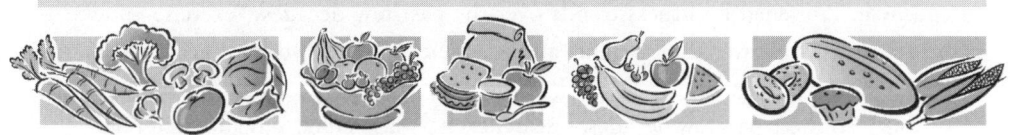

Regular exercise and physical activity are key parts of living well. Exercise is intrinsically linked with nutrition as two complementary sides of a healthy lifestyle. The food you eat represents the energy you take into your body, and your physical activity represents the energy you expend. Maintaining the two in balance is one of the most important tasks of staying healthy throughout life. The federal government's *Dietary Guidelines* and Food Guide Pyramid have recently been modified to reflect this growing recognition. In its newest incarnation, the pyramid has become a staircase representing the need for exercise—both to work off the energy taken in through food and to maintain health and prevent disease.

It's very common for women to have questions and confusions about exercise during pregnancy. Is it safe to exercise? Will vigorous activity hurt my baby? What kinds of activities are "off-limits" during pregnancy and when? With their bodies changing and suddenly feeling more fragile, many pregnant women worry that any physical exertion may harm their babies or put their pregnancy in jeopardy.

In fact, pregnant women can and should engage in regular physical activity. Unless you have a medical condition that puts exercise off-limits, engaging in regular physical activity during pregnancy is not only safe, it has some important benefits for your health. Even though your body may feel strange to you, it is still a fit and powerful body that needs movement and physical challenge to stay healthy. The trick is to modify the activities you choose for your new shape, your new needs, and the safety concerns of pregnancy.

What Is Exercise?

When most of us hear the word *exercise*, we think of working out at the gym, playing a vigorous sport, taking a long run or bike ride, or some other major physical endeavor. Propelled by fitness trends over the past few decades, "exercise" now brings up a whole world of weights and machines, classes, workout gear, sports drinks, and competition.

But over these past few decades, researchers have also come to realize that regular exercise—from thirty minutes to an hour most days a week—is the best way to stay healthy and ward off weight gain and chronic disease. Given our current connotation of the word *exercise*, these guidelines can seem daunting. Other than a celebrity with a personal trainer, who has time to go to the gym every day?

In fact, what matters for health is an active lifestyle. Because many people drive to work and sit most of the day, taking time to work out in sessions at the gym is sometimes the best way to build physical activity into their lifestyle. But someone who bikes to work, walks around the neighborhood to run errands, gardens in the backyard, and climbs three flights of stairs to an office or apartment a few times a day may not need as many prescribed bouts of exercise.

A better term to keep in mind is *physical activity*. What matters is how much you move your body every day and how much energy you expend. One person could eat just two or three large meals a day, while another person could snack all day, and both could wind up eating the same number of calories. Physical activity is similar: you might prefer "meals"—long, sustained periods of exercise—or you may be an activity "snacker," grabbing your exercise here and there. Either way, it's the total activity that counts for your overall health. The *Dietary Guidelines for Americans* recommend that, in the absence of medical or obstetric complications, pregnant women incorporate thirty minutes or more of moderate-intensity physical activity on most, if not all, days of the week. Try to aim for some periods of sustained activity, and on the days when you don't have much time, try to fit in several short walks or other exercises that add up to at least thirty minutes.

Different kinds of exercise have different effects on your body and carry different benefits. A good exercise program or active lifestyle includes some of each:

- *Cardiovascular* or *aerobic* exercise is the kind that raises your heart rate and makes you sweat and breathe faster. It challenges the ability of your cardiovascular and respiratory systems to supply your body with oxygen during sustained activity.
- *Muscular endurance* is the ability of your muscles to perform without fatigue. Many aerobic exercises and yoga postures involve muscular endurance.
- *Muscular strength* involves using your muscles to exert force against some form of resistance, whether it is weights or even just the force of gravity or the pull of water.
- *Flexibility* exercises aim to improve the range of motion around a joint. Good flexibility can prevent injuries and muscle stiffness.

Why Exercise in Pregnancy Is Different

During pregnancy, your body changes in several ways that can affect movement and physical activity. Some of these changes are simple mechanics. Your growing breasts become heavier and cause more discomfort than before. As your pregnancy progresses, the weight of your baby changes your center of gravity, making balance more challenging. The extra weight you carry puts greater stress on your joints. Your joints actually become more flexible and mobile—a phenomenon that probably helps the pubic bones of pregnant women accommodate the delivery of a baby—which can set the stage for injuries if flexibility is pushed too far.

In addition to the risk of injuries, exercise during pregnancy might also affect your baby's health through the physiological changes you experience, though these effects are not well understood. Pregnancy causes a woman's blood volume to expand, her heart to beat faster and pump more blood at each beat, and her metabolism to speed up—effects that are also caused by exercise. Some people have worried that strenuous exercise might interfere with the ability of a woman's body to protect and deliver nutrients to her fetus. So far, research has shown that regular, moderate exercise is safe during pregnancy.

As you exercise and perform physical activities, you may notice that your endurance decreases, that you become short of breath easier, and that your ability to move is hindered by the extra weight you carry. Once-familiar movements may need to be adjusted as your posture and body alignment change. Many women notice that their performance and enjoyment declines the most in weight-bearing exercises—those that involve carrying the weight of your body, such as running, hiking, or aerobics. It's important not to abandon physical activity altogether because of the changes you experience. Movement may feel different and less effortless than usual, but it's still important to find activities you like to do.

The Benefits of Exercise During Pregnancy

Exercise or regular physical activity may help offset some of the problems experienced during pregnancy, such as varicose veins, leg cramps, fatigue, and constipation. It can help maintain the muscle tone of your abdomen, uterus, and vagina and can help prevent urinary incontinence and lower back pain that are sometimes caused by pregnancy.

Physical activity, along with diet, is one of the factors that helps keep your metabolism running smoothly. Your metabolism is like the body's engine and includes all the systems and chemical reactions involved in taking energy from food and using it to fuel the body's activities and keep you alive. Many of the primary causes of death and disease stem from metabolic problems, including heart disease, diabetes, and obesity. Good nutrition and physical activity are the twin solutions to preventing these problems. When you're pregnant, your entire metabolic engine must be retooled to accommodate the needs of a growing baby. Pregnant women

Can Exercise Affect Your Baby?

In addition to the benefits that exercise can bring to you, physical activity may help improve the delivery of oxygen and nutrients to your baby. During cardiovascular exercise, your blood rushes away from the core of your body and out to working muscles and skin. During the period you are exercising, blood flow in the placenta actually decreases. However, studies have found that women who perform regular exercises can augment their body's delivery system—increasing blood and placenta volume and boosting the amount of blood their hearts can pump. One prospective randomized trial found that regular, weight-bearing exercise increased the volume and function of the placenta and slightly raised the birth weight of the baby. So regular exercise may actually help the placenta do its job, especially in later trimesters. The relationship between exercise and fetal development is complex, and so far we do not know how different exercises might affect a baby differently.

are more susceptible to metabolic problems such as high blood pressure and high blood sugar, and some of these problems may also affect the health of a growing fetus. By keeping this engine in good working condition, you can help prevent some of the metabolic complications of pregnancy.

Cardiovascular Exercise

Studies that have examined women who engage in fairly strenuous cardiovascular exercise have not found any detrimental effects on their babies. However, most of the exercise regimens recommended for pregnant women focus on slower exercises that avoid risk of injury or undue pressure on joints and the abdominal area. Exercises that don't involve carrying your own weight are easier to perform throughout your pregnancy, and they free you from worrying about maintaining your balance and posture. For any cardiovascular exercise, it's important to stay hydrated. Drink a glass of water before and after the exercise, and if possible, take small sips from a water bottle as you go. Pregnant women can engage in lots of different activities; these are some of the best and safest:

• *Walking.* Nothing beats walking for a low-impact activity that's easy to do and enjoyable. Whether you are simply walking in your neighborhood, near the office on a lunch break, or out in the woods for an easy hike, walking is the easiest way to add to your daily activity level. Walking for long periods of time can be difficult late in pregnancy, though, so it's good to have other non-weight-bearing options.

• *Swimming.* When you're in the water, your body is buoyant, which means you are temporarily relieved from the effects of gravity, including joint pressure from the extra weight you carry. Because you are supported by the water, there is no need to worry about falls or lack of balance because of your changing shape. Because it is the ultimate low-impact sport, swimming is a great activity during pregnancy. Just avoid diving or jumping into the water, and also avoid hot tubs, because the high temperatures may be harmful.

• *Water aerobics.* For those who are poor swimmers or don't like to do laps, many pools and gyms offer water aerobics classes that avoid all the stress and strain of working out on dry land.

• *Stationary bikes and low-impact cardiovascular machines.* You can use various low-impact machines at the gym, including elliptical trainers, which are easier on the joints than running. Stationary bikes are even better, because the weight of your body is supported while you move your legs.

• *Low-impact aerobics.* If possible, find a class that is geared toward expectant mothers or is listed as low-impact. In addition to gyms and fitness centers, many hospitals and health clinics offer special fitness classes for pregnant women. Otherwise, make sure your instructor knows you are pregnant, and ask for modifications of strenuous exercises. Avoid any jerking or bouncing movements, and don't push your limits just to follow along. You can also rent videos and DVDs of prenatal aerobics classes.

Stretches for Pregnancy

Stretching before and after a workout will help to prevent muscle injury and stiffness and promote better flexibility. Take the time to stretch your arms, legs, back, neck, and chest and shoulder area rather than just working on one or two areas. Stretching throughout the day, especially later in pregnancy, can help to relieve some of the discomfort your body may experience. For instance, stretching the arms, chest, and shoulder area can help to counteract the effects of slouching under the added weight of your breasts. And postures that help you align your spine correctly can help to offset the exaggerated hollow of your spine that may develop as your belly grows. Prenatal yoga is also a good way to incorporate stretching and muscular endurance into your routine.

Here is a simple series of stretches you can do at the beginning and end of the day, or any time you need a break:

• Sit on the floor with ankles crossed. Allow the knees to relax down toward the ground. You can deepen the stretch in your inner thighs by bringing the soles of the feet together. To help the inner-thigh muscles relax, cup your hands against the outer sides of your knees and push your knees downward toward the floor while resisting the force of your legs with your hands.

• Now extend your legs in front of you, keeping your feet apart. Keep your knees slightly bent if you feel tension in your hamstrings (the large muscles on the backs of your thighs). Gently lean forward as far as you can without pulling your hamstrings—it may be only an inch or two. make sure that you hinge at your hips with your spine straight, even if you only stretch a short distance. Repeat several times, holding a few seconds each time.

• Keeping your feet stretched in front of you, or returning to the easier ankles-crossed position, bend your elbows and place your hands gently on your shoulders. Move your elbows backward in slow circles to relieve tension in the shoulders and open your chest.

• Stretch your arms straight overhead, keeping your shoulder blades relaxed down rather than pulling the shoulder muscles up toward your neck. Slowly reach the right hand higher than the left, and then reach the left hand higher than the right. To deepen the stretch, bend toward the opposite side while reaching with your arm, making sure not to arch the lower back. This exercise will help relieve shoulder tightness and tension under the rib cage.

• For an additional postural awareness, perform these exercises with your back against a wall, using your abdominal muscles to bring as much of your back in contact with the wall as possible. Straighten your arms against the wall at shoulder level. Then bring your arms slowly upward, and hold the position for a few seconds.

Never move beyond your comfort level—stretching should never cause pain. Pregnant women may notice they are more flexible than before as their joints become looser in preparation for birth. This hypermobility can put you at risk of injury if you push your limits too far.

Muscle Rx

A woman's body becomes structurally stressed during pregnancy, as the weight of her child pulls on her spine and may force her lower back to hollow and her abdominal muscles to lengthen. By concentrating on strengthening the "core" muscles of your abdomen, lower back, and pelvic floor, you can help prevent some of the discomfort that comes from poor posture and alignment. These muscle exercises are not about keeping your body looking svelte during pregnancy, which is an impossibility anyway for most women as they naturally put on weight. The improvements will be felt rather than seen—focus on feeling healthy and strong.

Pelvic Floor Exercises

Many women are unaware of the muscles in their pelvic floor and the importance they have in pregnancy and immediately after. You can think of this sheet of muscles forming a floor or hammock, with your pubic bone at one end and your tailbone at the other. It includes the circular sphincter muscles that control your urethra, vagina, and anus. The pelvic floor supports your pelvic organs against any pressures on them, including the baby and forces of lifting. By exercising your pelvic muscles, you can help improve your delivery and prevent muscle weakness during pregnancy. A recent clinical trial found that pelvic floor exercises could prevent the urinary incontinence that some women experience after giving birth, even after a Cesarean section.

Pelvic floor contractions, also called Kegel exercises, are easy to do and, once you get the hang of them, can be done just about anywhere and any time. You can identify these invisible, internal muscles by starting and stopping your urine flow midstream (some people mistakenly use their thigh or buttock muscles, but these should remain relaxed). You can also try inserting a finger in your vagina when contracting—you should feel the walls of the vagina tighten. Try these exercises, which can be performed before, during, and after your pregnancy:

- *Pelvic floor contractions.* Practice contracting the pelvic muscles and holding for a few seconds, and then relax for ten seconds. Do three sets of ten contractions a day, aiming for a duration of ten seconds at each contraction.
- *The elevator.* Draw your pelvic muscles in and up a little at a time, imagining an elevator ascending higher and higher. Once you've reached your limit, slowly relax them, as if descending one floor at a time.

Abdominal Exercises

Strengthening the abdominal muscles during pregnancy can help you better support the weight of your baby and help your lower back stay aligned. The purpose of abdominal exercises is not to try to keep your tummy flat—the growth of your abdomen in pregnancy is unavoidable and absolutely necessary to accommodate your baby! Instead, the goal is to keep the muscles strong and supportive.

• *Pelvic tilts.* Moving the pelvis backward as if to flatten the curve of your lower back helps to work the abdominal muscles while relieving muscle stiffness and tension in the spine and promoting better alignment if done frequently. It can help counteract the tendency of the pelvis to shift forward during pregnancy, which enhances the curvature of the spine. Try performing the pelvic tilt illustrated in Figure 8.1.

Many people confuse this movement with the common "cat stretch," by rounding their shoulders and upper back. In this case, focus on the pelvis and lower back instead. Get on all fours, and tilt your pelvis down while pulling your abdominals in toward your spine. Hold for a few seconds, then relax back to a straight—or neutral—spine. Note: many yoga classes practice the opposite stretch—tilting the buttocks up and letting the spine sag to exaggerate the natural curve of the back. During pregnancy, you want to focus only on flattening the back or rounding it against its natural curve, which becomes more pronounced when you are pregnant. You can also practice this pose lying on your back with knees bent. Imagine your pelvis bones are a bowl and you are tilting the bowl back toward your head, flattening out the curve of your back against the floor. Again, focus only on flattening the curve of your back, *not* tilting the pelvis forward to exaggerate the curve.

• *Curl-ups.* It's important to strengthen your abdominal muscles during pregnancy, as they support your growing baby. Lie on your back with knees bent, and cross your arms over your chest. Take a deep breath in and as you exhale, bring your

Figure 8.1   The Pelvic Tilt

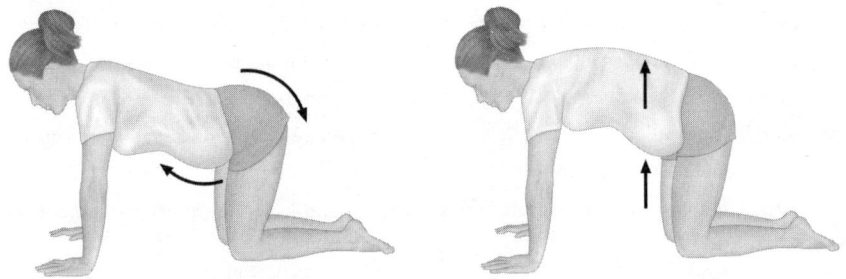

belly button toward your spine by tightening your abdominal muscles. Slowly curl your head and chest up a few inches off the ground, then lower them slowly. Do *not* raise the body completely to your knees. Alternate moving your body forward, bringing it diagonally to each knee. Repeat as many times as feels comfortable. You can deepen the exercise further by crossing your arms over your chest or, as you progress, placing your hands behind your head.

Some women experience a condition called *diastasis recti*, in which the central fibrous seam between the two sides of their abdominal muscles separate and bulging occurs at the midline. If you are performing a curl-up and notice a bulge or soft region more than three fingers in width between the taut central abdominals, you may have this condition, which can be worsened by performing abdominal exercises improperly. A knowledgeable trainer or yoga instructor can show you how to perform special abdominal exercises to help correct the condition—

Prenatal Yoga

Yoga classes have gone more and more mainstream in recent years, and many classes are now offered specifically for pregnant women. Yoga can be a great way to improve muscle strength, endurance, flexibility, and balance. Even though yoga has a reputation for relaxation, many styles of yoga can be physically demanding. It involves moving the body into positions that are challenging and potentially stressful on muscles and joints. It's important to find an instructor who is knowledgeable about the special concerns of pregnant women. Specialized prenatal yoga classes can be found in many yoga or maternity centers, and some teachers can work individually with pregnant women to modify poses in normal yoga classes.

Currently, there is no universal standard of certification for yoga instructors, though a group called Yoga Alliance has established a National Yoga Registry and recognizes qualified instructors as Certified Yoga Instructors who have completed either two hundred hours of training or five hundred hours of training. Training includes basic yoga technique, teaching time, and introduction to anatomy and physiology. Beyond that basic certification, yoga instructors can take a special course in prenatal yoga. If you are planning on taking a yoga class, spend some time finding out about the instructor of the class. Choose an instructor who has either completed certification and special course work on prenatal yoga or is a licensed personal trainer, physical therapist, or health-care professional and has a knowledge of the physical changes that take place in pregnancy and how they affect movement and exercise.

with curl-ups, for instance, it helps to place the hands against the sides of the abdominals and physically hold the muscles together or wrap a towel around your back and pull the ends together over your belly button as you curl up. Women with this condition should consult their doctor to diagnose and offer ways to correct the separation, which can also surface after delivery. Though it is not immediately dangerous, it may compromise the ability of your abdominal muscles to support your body.

For more specific muscle and postural exercises during pregnancy, see *Essential Exercises for the Childbearing Year*, 4th ed., by physical therapist Elizabeth Noble.

Exercises and Activities to Avoid

Your body is now a home to a quickly growing—and fragile—fetus. Because of this new role, during pregnancy you should take care to avoid any activities that could cause injury to your baby, such as these:

• Avoid activities that put you in danger of falling or receiving abdominal injury. Think contact sports (ice hockey, basketball, soccer), fast-paced or risky outdoor sports (downhill skiing, mountain biking), or activities that require fine coordination or new skills and carry a risk of injury if not performed correctly.

• Avoid any activity that could put pressure or force on your tummy area. This includes postures that involve lying on your stomach. Scuba diving is also out, because the intense pressure of deep water can harm your baby.

• Avoid vigorous, intense exercise. You may find that seemingly simple activities leave you feeling short of breath. You don't need to be afraid if an activity such as walking up a flight of stairs makes you breathe a little heavier than usual, but if you find you are struggling to breathe, slow down. Some health organizations advise not to let your heartbeat exceed 140 beats per minute. An easier guideline is that if you are too out of breath to carry on a conversation, you're exercising too hard.

• After the first trimester, avoid any vigorous exercises that involve lying on your back for very long, because the positioning and weight of your baby can interfere with proper blood circulation. For yoga and other postures that involve lying on the back, placing a rolled-up blanket or pillow under one side to tilt your body can help promote good circulation.

- Avoid activities in potentially dangerous conditions, such as very hot, humid weather or extreme cold.

- Avoid movements or postures that cause your pelvis to tilt backward and your lower spine to curve. For example, lifting both straightened legs off the ground while lying down puts too much stress on the lower back and abdominals.

- Avoid activities with bouncing or jolting movements, such as horseback riding or high-impact aerobics.

How to Exercise Safely

Dress for your intended activity. Wear comfortable shoes and clothing that lets you stay cool, and bring extra layers for cold-weather activities. You may need to use a more supportive sports bra if your breasts feel heavy or tender. Bring a bottle of water with you, and take short, frequent drinks to stay hydrated.

Before you begin any aerobic exercise, start by stretching and warming up gradually for about five minutes before you exercise. Aim for a twenty- to thirty-minute low-impact, low-intensity session of aerobic exercise. If you are planning activities that last any longer than that—for instance, an afternoon hike or a long gardening session—take breaks during the activity and make sure you have a snack available to keep your blood sugar from dipping. After your session, try to take a full fifteen minutes for a cooldown, including light stretches, relaxation, and breathing exercises to help loosen your muscles.

Slowing Down

Relaxation and breathing exercises can be a good way to cool down after exercise, prevent muscle tightness, and ward off stress. Try lying down or sitting comfortably in a chair and taking a few minutes to mentally scan your body beginning with your toes and working your way up to your face, relaxing each part as you focus on it. You can also try breathing slowly, inhaling for three or four counts, holding the breath for the same number of counts, and then exhaling for twice the number of counts. Take the air deep into your lungs, as if you were breathing into your belly, rather than taking shallow breaths only into your chest.

If you were very sedentary before pregnancy, now is a good opportunity to start building more physical activity into your day—by walking more, visiting the gym more regularly, or taking yoga classes. But now is *not* the time to try to master a new sport, push your performance, or suddenly launch a vigorous exercise regimen. Many women find they can safely exercise strenuously in pregnancy, but only if their bodies were conditioned to begin with. Work within your established level of conditioning, and instead aim for more regularity.

The American College of Obstetricians and Gynecologists lists these warning signs to be alert to. If you experience any of these symptoms, stop exercising and call your doctor:

- Pain
- Vaginal bleeding
- Dizziness or faintness
- Increased shortness of breath
- Rapid heartbeat
- Difficulty walking
- Uterine contractions and chest pain
- Abnormal fluid leaking from the vagina

Women who have a history of difficult pregnancies or certain medical conditions may need to limit their activity, especially after the first trimester. It's a good idea to have a discussion with your doctor about your intended exercise level early in pregnancy.

Physical Activity During Pregnancy: The Bottom Line

You can and should remain physically active during pregnancy. Physical activity can help your metabolism run smoothly, help relieve discomforts of pregnancy, and keep you feeling strong and healthy. Keep the following in mind:

- A good activity should include cardiovascular exercise, muscle strength, muscle endurance, and flexibility.
- Pregnant women need to modify their activities to keep from putting stress on their abdominal area and lower back, to avoid injury and discomfort, and

to accommodate the changes in posture and balance that come with pregnancy.

- Physical activity should be a regular and frequent part of your life. Choose the kinds of activities that fit your lifestyle, whether it is short frequent walks throughout the day, scheduled classes, or regular visits to the gym. What matters is how your activity level adds up day to day and week to week.

The Active Lifestyle

If you find it difficult to take the time or maintain the energy for regular exercise sessions or planned activities, you can find other ways to make your lifestyle a more active one and receive the benefits of physical activity.

- Get a pedometer. These small devices, which you can wear on your waistband, can tell you how many steps you are taking throughout the day. They can help you set goals and check your progress. You'll be surprised how building a few short walks into your day can add up to miles. A good goal for adults is to walk ten thousand steps a day most days of the week. Pregnant women can adjust their goals to a comfortable level depending on their stage of pregnancy.

- Make walking part of your commute. If you are going to work every day, try to build a little more walking into your commute. If you drive to work, this might mean parking farther away than you usually do.

- Take walking breaks. Make time for some short walks throughout your day, even if it's just a quick walk around the block or around the building at work. Walking after eating a meal can also help relieve digestive discomfort.

- Make physical activity social. Meet your friends for a short social walk or a visit to the gym rather than sitting down at a café.

- Take the stairs instead of the escalator or elevator. Get in the habit of looking for the stairs at shopping malls or other buildings you frequent. Stair climbing can become more difficult toward the end of your pregnancy, so don't push your comfort level.

- Clean up. Doing housework, gardening, and taking care of the home can burn a lot of calories. But take care to avoid jobs that require breathing strong fumes, such as painting, and keep rooms well ventilated. Wash hands after gardening outdoors.

9

Recipes and Meal Planning

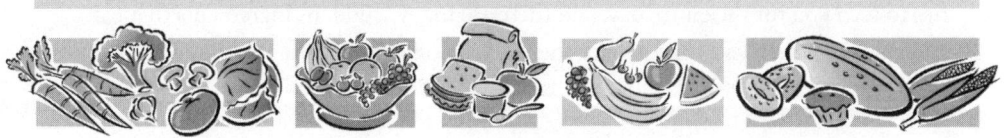

N ow that we've talked about some fundamentals of good nutrition, here are some specific recipes and tips for putting what you've learned into practice. The recipes are designed to provide nutrition that pregnant women need, but they are also delicious and nutritious options for the rest of your family, as well as beyond pregnancy.

Power Snacks

Most typical snack foods are high in simple carbohydrates and fats but low in proteins, vitamins, and minerals. Try to put snacks together that pair healthy carbohydrates from fruits, vegetables, and whole grains with a food high in protein. This will give you long-lasting energy and important nutrients. These are some examples:

- Fruit wedges with ½ cup of low-fat cottage cheese or yogurt
- Raw vegetables with hummus
- Fruit with one ounce of low-fat cheese, such as mozzarella string cheese
- Fruit or vegetable pieces with ¼ cup nuts

- Natural peanut butter (no hydrogenated oils) spread on a slice of whole-grain bread or whole-grain trans fat–free crackers
- Peanut butter spread on celery sticks or apple wedges

The Ins and Outs of Eating Out

Dining out can be one of the major contributors of excess calories, unhealthy fats, and sugars in our diet. Portion sizes at restaurants may now contain enough calories to feed you for the entire day, and there are many "hidden" ingredients that can add calories where you least expect them. Here are some tips for eating out:

Making Healthy Food Convenient

Eating two or three small snacks throughout the day between meals can help to keep your blood sugar from dipping too low and, if the snacks are healthy ones, add important nutrients to your diet. Unfortunately, many of the most convenient snacks are filled with trans and saturated fat, sugar, and excess salt, with little real nourishment. Keep a few healthier snacks with you during the day to prevent unhealthy snacking. These are a few accessories that help make healthy foods convenient:

- **Small plastic bags.** Use these to portion out sliced vegetables and fruits, berries, nuts, whole-grain crackers free of trans fats, and other snack foods. Keep a few of these pre-filled in the fridge or on your kitchen shelves so you can grab and go.

- **Small lidded plastic containers.** Storage containers now come in extra-small sizes perfect for keeping dipping sauces such as hummus, peanut butter, and low-fat cream cheese. You can also premix your own yogurt or cottage cheese with fruit, nuts, or berries, which is healthier than buying the small containers of sweetened flavored yogurt.

- **Insulated lunch bag or small cooler.** These can help keep perishable foods cool during the day if you are out running errands or don't have access to a fridge.

- **Insulated thermos.** Use a thermos to carry homemade soups such as the Ginger Butternut Squash Soup in this chapter, or cold liquids such as skim milk.

- *Don't start out starving.* Skipping meals or avoiding food before a meal out can cause you to overeat once you're at the restaurant. Plan to eat a light snack before dining out for dinners, realizing that traveling to the restaurant, waiting for a table, reading the menu, and ordering all add to your wait time before you eat. Have a piece of fruit, some vegetable slices, a handful of crackers, or a small handful of nuts beforehand.

- *Make requests.* Don't be afraid to ask how a particular dish is prepared, and request healthier ways of cooking—for instance, baking or broiling chicken instead of frying. Many restaurants will gladly serve meals with steamed vegetables or a small salad instead of french fries or other unhealthier foods.

- *Bring it home.* At many restaurants these days, a reasonable portion may be half or even less than what you are served. Make it a habit to leave enough food for lunch the next day, and take it home with you. If you find you are still hungry, you can always finish the meal later.

- *Think small.* If eating only half your meal all the time requires too much self-control for you, try to order smaller items off the menu, such as appetizers, side dishes, and à la carte items. But be careful—not every appetizer is necessarily

Eating Tip for Morning Sickness

Women who experience nausea or vomiting during their pregnancies (often called "morning sickness," though it can strike at any time of the day!) may find that the smell of cooking and hot foods turns them off. Other women simply feel an aversion to strong food smells. You may find that cold foods that don't require cooking are much easier to prepare and eat. This chapter includes several cold recipes that can help you choose healthy foods that don't make you feel sick, including Roasted Beet, Baby Spinach, and Goat Cheese Salad (substitute canned beets instead of cooking them yourself) with Walnut Vinaigrette; Eda-Mommy (Edamame) Vegetable Salad with Vegetable Vinaigrette; Peach Yogurt Smoothie; Chocolate Fondue (for dipping fruits or soy pretzels); Strawberry, Banana, Yogurt, and Muesli Parfait; Strawberry Tofu "Ice Cream"; Quinoa Salad with Apricots and Pistachios; and Fruit Soup.

smaller than a main dish. For instance, a big plate of nachos at a Mexican restaurant will have more calories and fat than a taco or enchilada à la carte with a side of beans.

• *Say no to nibbling.* Once you start feeling full, avoid the urge to keep nibbling at your food. Have the waitperson take your plate away once you feel you've had enough.

• *Take your time.* Eating too fast can cause you to overeat, because it takes fifteen to twenty minutes for your body to know it's full. If you are out with others, take time to enjoy the conversation. If you're dining alone, bring a book or newspaper to encourage yourself to linger.

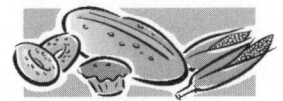 **Recipes**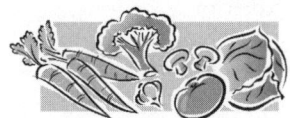

Zucchini Bread

This is a good source of essential fatty acids and fiber.

1 large or 2 small ripe bananas
2 high-omega eggs
1 teaspoon vanilla extract
¼ cup olive or canola oil
1 cup grated zucchini
½ cup oat bran
¾ cup whole wheat flour
½ cup ground flaxseeds
¾ cup (3 ounces) walnut pieces
½ cup (4 ounces) raisins
½ teaspoon salt
½ teaspoon baking powder
½ teaspoon baking soda
½ teaspoon cinnamon

Makes one 9" × 5" loaf pan or twelve 2½ inch muffins.

Preheat oven to 350°F. Prepare loaf pan or muffin tins with cooking spray, or coat with a little oil and dusting of flour.

In a blender or food processor, puree bananas. Gradually add eggs and vanilla. Beat until smooth. Gradually add oil. Pour into bowl with grated zucchini.

In a separate bowl combine everything else. Add the flour mixture to the banana mixture, and mix and blend thoroughly. Pour into prepared pan or muffin tins. Bake approximately 45minutes for the loaf pan or 25 minutes for muffins. Bake until toothpick inserted in center comes out dry.

Ginger Butternut Squash Soup

This is rich in vitamin A.

2 tablespoons olive oil
1 large onion, diced
3 carrots, peeled and sliced
2 tablespoons peeled and chopped ginger
1 large butternut squash (approximately 4 to 5 pounds), peeled, seeded,
   and cut into 1- to 2-inch pieces
1 teaspoon cinnamon
1 48-ounce can low-sodium chicken or vegetable stock
1½ teaspoons coconut extract
1½ cups 1 percent milk
Salt and pepper, to taste

Makes approximately 10 to 12 cups, depending on size of squash.

Place olive oil in large pot on medium heat, and sauté onion until translucent. Add carrots and ginger and cook for 3 to 5 more minutes on medium to low heat. Add squash, cinnamon, stock, coconut extract, and milk. Simmer on low for approximately 30 to 40 minutes or until squash and carrots are soft. Remove from heat. Let cool slightly and puree in blender or food processor. Season with salt and pepper to taste.

Sweet Roasted Garlic and White Bean Dip

This is high in fiber, folate, and protein and is a great snack.

5 large cloves garlic, peeled
½ cup olive oil (save after cooking for Whole Wheat Dipping Chips,
    recipe follows)
1 15-ounce can cannellini beans (white kidney beans)
½ cup vegetable or tomato juice
Salt and pepper, to taste

Makes approximately 1 ¼ cups.

Preheat oven to 350°F. Place garlic cloves in a small, ovenproof container; cover garlic with oil. Cover with foil and place in oven for approximately 40 minutes or until garlic is soft when pressed with a fork. Remove soft garlic, and save oil. Rinse and drain beans. Place drained beans in blender or food processor with cooked garlic, and puree until smooth. Gradually add vegetable juice and 1 tablespoon of reserved oil; add salt and pepper to taste. Serve with Whole Wheat Dipping Chips or multigrain crackers and/or raw vegetables for dipping.

Whole Wheat Dipping Chips

Here is a great alternative to fried chips for dipping. These chips provide fiber and the olive oil provides essential fatty acid.

½ 8-ounce package whole wheat pita bread (without partially
    hydrogenated oils)
Reserved oil from roasting garlic or ½ cup olive oil
Sea salt and freshly ground pepper, to taste

Makes 4 servings.

Preheat oven to 300°F. Slice pita bread in half, and brush each side with reserved garlic oil. Cut into wedges and place on sheet pan. Sprinkle with salt and pepper. Place in oven for approximately 5 minutes or until crispy.

Whole Wheat and Flax Soda Bread

This is rich in omega-3 and fiber.

1 cup ground flaxseeds (grind in coffee grinder)
1 cup oat bran
2 cups whole wheat flour
Zest of 1 orange
½ cup sugar
1 tablespoon baking powder
1 teaspoon baking soda
¼ teaspoon salt
1 cup raisins (optional)
½ cup walnuts or almonds (optional)
1 high-omega egg
1 cup low-fat buttermilk

Makes one loaf.

Preheat oven to 350°F. Combine ground flaxseeds, oat bran, whole wheat flour, orange zest, sugar, baking powder, baking soda, salt, raisins, and nuts.

Beat egg with buttermilk, pour into dry mixture, and mix until blended. Press into greased loaf pan, or shape into round loaf approximately 8 inches in diameter by 1¼ inches deep and place on greased cookie pan. Bake approximately 40 minutes.

Barley Breakfast Cereal

This is a good source of fiber and niacin.

    1 cup low-fat milk
    ½ cup quick-cooking Quaker Barley
    1 tablespoon maple syrup
    2 tablespoons raisins
    ¼ teaspoon cinnamon
    2 tablespoons chopped almonds or walnuts

Makes two ¾-cup servings.

Bring milk to a boil and stir in barley, maple syrup, raisins, cinnamon, and nuts. Simmer on low heat for 10 minutes. Remove from heat and let sit covered for 5 minutes; stir and serve.

Tofu Chili

This is high in antioxidants, protein, folate, vitamin C, and potassium and low in saturated fat.

1 14-ounce container firm tofu
2 tablespoons canola oil
1 small onion, diced
2 cloves garlic, peeled and sliced
1 green pepper, seeded and diced
2 teaspoons ground cumin
2 teaspoons chili powder
1 teaspoon dried cilantro
1 tablespoon Worcestershire sauce
1 28-ounce can diced tomatoes (make sure no sugar added)
1 1-pound 13-ounce can red kidney beans
1 large ripe avocado

Makes 6 ½ cups.

Freeze tofu in container, defrost, drain liquid off, and crumble to resemble ground meat. Place oil in large saucepan, and sauté onion, garlic, and pepper until onion is translucent. Add cumin, chili powder, cilantro, Worcestershire sauce, tomatoes, and beans. Simmer on low heat 20 minutes. Add crumbled tofu and simmer 20 minutes more; remove from heat. Cut avocado into ½-inch pieces and fold in before serving.

Serve with Brown Basmati Rice with Ground Flax (see recipe).

Brown Basmati Rice with Ground Flax

This is high in omega-3 fats and fiber.

½ small onion, diced
1 small red pepper, diced
1 tablespoon canola oil
½ cup uncooked brown basmati rice
1½ cups low-sodium chicken or vegetable stock (or water with low-
    sodium bouillon cube)
1 bay leaf
¼ cup ground flaxseeds (grind in coffee grinder)
1 bunch scallions, sliced (white part with a little green)

Makes approximately 2 cups cooked rice.

Sauté onion and pepper in oil over low heat until soft. Add rice, stock, and bay leaf. Cover and simmer approximately 45 minutes. Remove from heat and let sit, covered, 5 more minutes. Remove bay leaf, stir in ground flax and sliced scallions, and serve.

Tilapia Tapenade

This is a good source of protein and antioxidants, including vitamin C.

1 pound boneless tilapia fillets
Salt and pepper, to taste
2 tablespoons olive oil
3 cloves garlic, sliced
1 red pepper, seeded and julienned
2 tablespoons capers
1 6-ounce jar marinated artichoke hearts (marinade should not include hydrogenated oils)
4–6 ounces quality pitted olives (Nicoise, Gaeta, country mix)
1 14½-ounce can diced tomatoes (no added sugar)
2 tablespoons lemon juice
4 large basil leaves, chopped

Makes two to three servings.

Preheat oven to 350°F. Sprinkle tilapia fillets with salt and pepper. Heat olive oil in large sauté pan. Place tilapia fillets in pan and cook 2 to 3 minutes on each side (so that color turns from opaque to white). Remove from pan and transfer to ovenproof dish. Place in oven to finish cooking and keep warm while preparing sauce. Place sliced garlic in pan and sauté until translucent. Add julienned red pepper, capers, artichoke hearts, olives, tomatoes, lemon juice, and basil. Simmer on low heat 5 minutes. Season with salt and pepper. Place fish fillets on plate, and spoon sauce over each fillet.

Roasted Beet, Baby Spinach, and Goat Cheese Salad

Beets are a good source of vitamin A, vitamin C, and folacin. Spinach is iron-rich, and walnuts are high in omega-6 and omega-3 fats.

3 ounces baby spinach
12–16 ounces fresh beets
1 tablespoon canola or olive oil
2–3 ounces pasteurized goat cheese, crumbled
2 ounces walnuts

Makes two servings.

Preheat oven to 350°F. Wash and dry baby spinach. Wash and cut off root ends and stems from beets, and toss with oil. Place beets in baking dish, cover with foil, and place in oven. Bake until a fork easily pierces each, approximately 30 to 40 minutes, depending on size of beets. Let cool and peel skins off. Dice and marinate in ¼ cup Walnut Vinaigrette (see recipe). Toss spinach with walnut dressing; add beets and goat cheese. Top with walnuts.

Walnut Vinaigrette

This is rich in omega-3 and omega-6 fats, and the orange juice helps the body absorb the iron from the spinach.

¼ cup orange juice
2 tablespoons cider vinegar
1 teaspoon salt
½ cup walnut oil

Makes ¾ cup.

Place orange juice, cider vinegar, and salt in blender. Blend until smooth. Slowly drizzle in walnut oil. Cover and refrigerate.

Dutch Banana Pancake

This is a very light textured pancake with fiber and omega fatty acids; it also has more protein than most pancakes.

½ cup whole wheat flour
1 tablespoon sugar
½ teaspoon salt
4 tablespoons walnuts
¼ teaspoon cinnamon
2 tablespoons protein powder (optional)
4 high-omega eggs
½ teaspoon vanilla extract
⅔ cup low-fat milk
4 tablespoons melted butter
2 ripe bananas

Makes four servings (¼ pancake).

Preheat oven to 400°F. Combine flour, sugar, salt, walnuts, cinnamon, and protein powder (if using). In a separate bowl, beat eggs until frothy, and add vanilla and milk. Add milk mixture to flour mixture and beat smooth. Add 2 tablespoons of the melted butter and mix well. Use rest of melted butter for cooking pancakes.

Pour a little butter in 9- to 10-inch ovenproof sauté pan, and slice all of the bananas into pan. Sauté briefly, and pour batter over bananas. Cook on top of stove just until edges of batter start to set, and then place in preheated oven for approximately 6 to 7 minutes. Cut into portions. Repeat with any remaining bananas and batter. Serve with Maple Yogurt (see recipe).

Variation: when in season, replace bananas with fresh blueberries (very high in antioxidants), and add some grated lemon zest in place of the cinnamon for a great pancake.

Maple Yogurt

A low-sugar alternative to maple syrup with the added protein of yogurt.

1 cup plain low-fat yogurt
2–3 tablespoons maple syrup
1 teaspoon vanilla
1 teaspoon ground cinnamon

Makes 1 cup.

Combine yogurt, maple syrup, vanilla, and cinnamon. Serve with Dutch Banana Pancake (see recipe) or over fresh fruit. This is also great as a dip with sliced apples.

Black Bean Dip with Tahini

This is rich in protein, folate, essential fatty acids, and fiber.

1 15½-ounce can black beans
1 tablespoon chopped fresh cilantro
1 small bunch scallions, chopped (white part only)
2 tablespoons lemon juice
½ cup tahini

Makes 1 cup.

Drain and rinse beans. Combine cilantro, scallions, lemon juice, and tahini. Roughly mash beans in food processor or blender. Add tahini mixture. Mix until blended. Use as a dip for raw vegetables and whole wheat pita chips or crackers made with no trans fats.

Mango and Avocado Chutney

This is rich in vitamin A and copper.

1 ripe mango
1 ripe avocado
1 small red pepper
1 tablespoon chopped fresh cilantro
2 tablespoons lemon juice
2 tablespoons walnut oil
½ teaspoon ground cumin
½ teaspoon salt

Makes approximately 3 cups.

Peel and dice mango and avocado. Seed and dice pepper. Add chopped cilantro, lemon juice, walnut oil, cumin, and salt. Toss together and chill. Serve over baked chicken or grilled fish.

Almond-Crusted Baked Chicken Breast

This is a good source of protein.

¾–1 pound boneless and skinless chicken breasts
Salt and pepper to taste
1 tablespoon Dijon mustard
1 cup almond meal (or 1 cup sliced almonds blended in coffee grinder)

Makes two servings.

Preheat oven to 350°F. Trim any fat off chicken breasts. Cover with plastic wrap and pound to approximately ½ original thickness. Sprinkle with salt and pepper; spread mustard on both sides of chicken, and dredge in almond meal. Place on sheet pan and place in oven. Bake approximately 20 minutes or until chicken is completely white when cut into. Top with Mango and Avocado Chutney (see recipe).

Collard Green Casserole

This is rich in vitamin A and folate.

1 16-ounce bag frozen chopped collard greens
2 cloves garlic
1 large shallot
2 tablespoons olive oil
½ package Neufchâtel cheese (⅓ less-fat or low-fat cream cheese)
1 tablespoon lemon juice
Salt and pepper, to taste

Makes 2 cups.

Preheat oven to 350°F. Run collard greens under water to defrost and squeeze out any excess water. Chop garlic and shallot and sauté in olive oil on medium-low heat until translucent. Remove from heat and stir in Neufchâtel cheese, collard greens, and lemon juice; season to taste with salt and pepper. Place in ovenproof pan and bake for 20 minutes or until hot.

Eda-Mommy (Edamame) Vegetable Salad

This is high in fiber and protein.

2 cups frozen shelled edamame
1 large red bell pepper
½ large bulb fennel
1 cup grated carrot
2 tablespoons chopped fresh parsley
1 bunch scallions, sliced (white part only)

Makes approximately 6 cups.

Bring 4 cups water to a boil and add edamame. Return to a boil and cook 5 minutes. Drain and cool. Dice pepper and fennel. Combine pepper, fennel, carrot, parsley, and scallions with edamame. Toss with Vegetable Vinaigrette (see recipe) and chill.

Vegetable Vinaigrette

With a lower ratio of fat to acid than typical dressings, this makes a "lighter" version of traditional vinaigrettes.

¼ cup vegetable juice (V8 or similar)
1 tablespoon tarragon vinegar
1 tablespoon lemon juice
½ cup olive oil
Salt and pepper, to taste

Makes approximately 1 cup.

Place vegetable juice, tarragon vinegar, and lemon juice in blender. Blend together. While blending, slowly add olive oil; season with salt and pepper to taste.

Peach Yogurt Smoothie

This is a good source of protein and calcium.

¾ cup fresh or frozen peaches (thawed)
½ cup plain low-fat yogurt
½ teaspoon vanilla
¼ teaspoon cinnamon
1 tablespoon orange juice concentrate

Makes one serving.

Place all ingredients in blender and puree until smooth. (Note: frozen peaches will create a "frozen yogurt" texture.)

Ginger Peppermint Tea

This soothes upset stomachs. Drink warm or chilled.

1 bunch fresh mint leaves
1½-inch piece fresh ginger
Honey, to taste

Makes 4 cups.

Wash and slice mint leaves and place in pot. Thinly slice ginger and add to mint in pot. Cover with 4 cups of water. Bring to a boil and lower heat. Simmer 15 minutes. Strain and sweeten with honey to taste. Serve hot or cold.

Tofu Tomato Sauce

Tomatoes are rich in antioxidants, and tofu contains plenty of protein, calcium, and B vitamins.

8 cloves garlic

3 tablespoons olive oil

2 28-ounce cans ground peeled tomatoes (organic if possible; no additives or added sugar)

1 tablespoon dried oregano

1 14-ounce package firm tofu, frozen and thawed (to create ground-beef-like texture)

2 tablespoons chopped fresh basil

Makes approximately 6 cups.

Slice garlic and sauté in olive oil in large pot on low heat until translucent. Add tomatoes and oregano. Simmer on low for 40 minutes.

Remove any "foam" that forms on the top. Stir occasionally. Crumble defrosted tofu and add to sauce after 40 minutes. Continue to simmer on low for 20 more minutes. Remove from heat and stir in basil. For a smoother sauce, puree in blender or food processor. Serve over whole wheat pasta or Barilla Plus pasta, which contains added protein, fiber, and omega-3 fatty acids.

Chocolate Fondue

Use for dipping fruits and soy pretzels, which are high in protein, fiber, and calcium.

6 ounces 70 percent bittersweet chocolate
3 ounces low-fat milk
¾ cup low-fat plain yogurt
2 tablespoons orange juice concentrate
1 tablespoon maple syrup
1 teaspoon vanilla extract

Makes 1¾ cups.

Cut chocolate into small pieces and melt in double boiler or in pot over hot water. Heat milk until very warm to the touch but not boiling and add to melted chocolate. Add yogurt, orange juice concentrate, maple syrup, and vanilla, and stir together over hot water until blended. Remove from heat and cool. Suggested fruits for dipping are mangos, strawberries, bananas, pineapple, and peaches.

Spinach (or Broccoli) and Cheddar "Quiche Cups"

These are a good source of protein, omega-3 fats, calcium, and iron.

1 10-ounce package (2 cups) frozen chopped spinach or broccoli
6 high-omega eggs
½ cup low-fat milk
1 tablespoon Dijon mustard
1½ cups shredded 2 percent reduced-fat sharp cheddar cheese

Makes 12 muffin "cups."

Preheat oven to 350°F. Defrost and drain extra water from spinach (or broccoli). Beat eggs with milk and mustard. Pour over drained spinach (or broccoli). Mix in cheddar cheese. Prepare muffin tin with cooking spray. Pour mixture into pan and bake 30 to 35 minutes until center of "muffin" is set.

Strawberry, Banana, Yogurt, and Muesli Parfait

This is a good source of calcium, protein, fiber, and vitamin C.

1 pint strawberries
1 ripe banana
1½ cups plain low-fat yogurt
½ teaspoon vanilla
½ teaspoon cinnamon
2 tablespoons maple syrup
1 cup muesli

Makes three servings.

Wash and remove stems from strawberries. Slice strawberries and bananas. Combine yogurt, vanilla, cinnamon, and maple syrup. Layer muesli, yogurt, bananas, and strawberries in three parfait or wine glasses, finishing with a layer of muesli.

Turkey and Broccoli Pasta Salad

This is high in protein, vitamin C, calcium, and fiber.

2 cups broccoli florets
4 cups water
1 pound turkey cutlets
1 tablespoon salt
Salt and pepper to taste
1 cup Barilla Plus penne pasta
½ 12-ounce jar roasted sweet red peppers
1 cup Tofu Ranch Dressing (see recipe)

Makes 5 cups.

Preheat oven to 350°F. Wash and cut broccoli florets. Bring water to a boil with 1 tablespoon salt, and add broccoli. Cook until fork-tender—approximately 3 to 5 minutes. Drain and run under cold water to stop the cooking process. Sprinkle turkey cutlets with salt and pepper, and place in cookie pan or in oven-proof pan. Bake approximately 10 to 15 minutes or until turkey is completely white when sliced into. Cool and cut into medium-size dice. Cook pasta in boiling water approximately 10 to 12 minutes. Drain and cool. Cut peppers into medium dice. Combine diced turkey, broccoli, roasted peppers, and pasta in large bowl. Toss with Tofu Ranch Dressing. This can be served hot or cold.

Tofu Ranch Dressing

This dressing is high in protein and healthy fats.

1 cup silken (soft) tofu
½ cup red wine vinegar
¼ cup walnut oil
¼ cup canola oil
1 large shallot, chopped
1 teaspoon dried parsley
1 teaspoon onion powder
1 teaspoon Worcestershire sauce
½ teaspoon granulated garlic
½ teaspoon salt
1 teaspoon Tabasco

Makes 2 cups.

Place tofu and vinegar in blender or food processor. Drizzle in walnut and canola oils while blending. Add remaining ingredients, and blend until smooth.

Mediterranean Tuna Salad

This is high in protein, omega-3 fats, vitamin C, and fiber.

3 ounces baby arugula
1 6-ounce can light tuna packed in water
½ 12-ounce jar roasted sweet red peppers
1 6-ounce jar marinated artichoke hearts (with no hydrogenated oils)
1 large ripe avocado
½ cup Balsamic Vinaigrette (see recipe)
3–4 ounces oil-cured or Kalamata olives

Makes two servings.

Wash and dry arugula. Drain water from tuna and peppers, and drain oil from artichoke hearts. Cut artichoke hearts in half. Dice avocado into medium cubes. Toss arugula with Balsamic Vinaigrette and divide between two salad bowls. Spoon tuna down the center of each bowl, followed by artichoke hearts, peppers, olives, and avocado.

Balsamic Vinaigrette

Another light, flavorful vinaigrette.

½ cup balsamic vinegar
1 tablespoon Dijon mustard
½ teaspoon salt
1 teaspoon dried basil or 1 tablespoon chopped fresh basil
1 cup olive or canola oil
Pepper, to taste

Makes 1½ cups.

Place vinegar, mustard, salt, and basil in blender. While blending, slowly add oil until smooth. Season with pepper to taste.

Strawberry Tofu "Ice Cream"

This is a good source of calcium, protein, vitamin C, and fiber.

¼ 14-ounce package firm tofu
1 cup frozen strawberries (no sugar added)
½ teaspoon vanilla
1 tablespoon honey or maple syrup
¼–⅓ cup soy milk or low-fat milk
¼ cup muesli

Makes one serving.

Place tofu, strawberries, vanilla, and honey or syrup in food processor or blender, and blend until smooth. While blending, add just enough milk to help blend smoothly. Remove from blender and top with muesli.

Curried Egg Salad

This is rich in omega-3 fats, protein, vitamin E, and choline.

4 high-omega eggs
1 large Granny Smith apple
2 heads endive (optional)
1 teaspoon curry powder
½ cup Tofu Ranch Dressing (see recipe)
1 ounce golden raisins
Whole wheat pita pockets (optional; make sure brand contains no
    partially hydrogenated oils)

Makes 2 cups.

Place eggs in saucepan and cover with cold water. Bring to a boil and remove from heat. Cover and let sit for 12 minutes. Run under cold water and remove shells. While eggs are cooking, cut apple into small dice. Cut bottom off of endive, if using. Pull leaves off; wash and dry. Mix curry powder into Tofu Ranch Dressing. When eggs are cool, cut into small pieces and mix together with diced apple, raisins, and curried tofu dressing. Spoon onto endive leaves, or put in whole wheat pita pockets.

Quinoa Salad with Apricots and Pistachios

This is rich in protein, magnesium, potassium, vitamin A, vitamin C, beta-carotene, and iron.

½ cup quinoa
½ cup diced dried apricots
½ cup pistachios
4 scallions, sliced
½ cup Tofu Ranch Dressing (see recipe)

Makes approximately 3 ½ cups.

Before cooking, rinse and drain quinoa with cold water until water runs clear. Place quinoa and 1 cup of water in saucepan and bring to a boil. Reduce to a simmer; cover and cook until all water is absorbed (10 to 15 minutes). When done the grain looks soft and translucent, and the germ ring will be visible along the outside edge of the grain. Let cool. Add apricots, pistachios, and scallions. Toss with Tofu Ranch Dressing.

Pumpkin and Quinoa Pudding

This is rich in vitamin A, protein, magnesium, potassium, and fiber.

¾ cup pumpkin puree
1 teaspoon vanilla extract
2 tablespoons orange juice concentrate
1 teaspoon pumpkin pie spice
¼ cup pure maple syrup
1 cup low-fat plain yogurt
1½ cups cooked quinoa
¼ cup walnuts (optional)

Makes 2¾ cups.

Combine pumpkin, vanilla, orange juice concentrate, pumpkin pie spice, and maple syrup. Stir in yogurt, and then stir in quinoa. Stir in walnuts last.

Trail Mix

This is rich in protein, folate, calcium, magnesium, potassium, vitamin A, and fiber.

1 cup old-fashioned oats
Zest of 1 orange
1 cup sliced almonds
¼ cup honey
½ cup (3 ounces) raisins
½ cup (3 ounces) shelled peanuts
½ cup dried apricots, cut into small pieces

Makes 3 cups.

Preheat oven to 350°F. Combine oats, orange zest, and almonds. Place on ungreased sheet pan, and place in oven for 15 minutes. Place toasted oats and almonds in bowl, and mix in honey. Grease sheet pan and crumble honey oats mixture onto pan; put back in oven for approximately 10 minutes or until golden. Cool and mix with raisins, peanuts, and apricots.

Peanut Buckwheat Noodles

These are a good source of protein.

½ cup natural peanut butter, smooth or chunky (no sugar added)
2 tablespoons sesame oil
1 tablespoon low-sodium soy sauce
3 tablespoons rice vinegar
1 teaspoon hot sauce
1 8.8-ounce package soba noodles (Japanese buckwheat pasta)
1 bunch scallions, sliced

Makes four servings.

Combine peanut butter, sesame oil, soy sauce, vinegar, hot sauce, and ½ cup hot of water. Mix until smooth. Cook soba noodles in boiling water 6 to 8 minutes. Drain noodles; rinse under cold water if serving cold. Toss with peanut dressing, and sprinkle with scallions.

Variation: add cooked chicken or vegetables to noodles with dressing or use peanut sauce over cooked chicken in a salad.

Lentil Soup

This is high in protein, fiber, folacin, phosphorus, potassium, iron, and vitamin A.

½ cup wild rice
3 tablespoons canola oil
3 cloves garlic, chopped
1 cup small diced carrots
1 cup small diced fennel
1 cup small diced onion
1½ cups lentils
2 teaspoons dried thyme
2 teaspoons ground cumin
2 bay leaves
2 32-ounce containers chicken or vegetable broth

Makes 9 cups.

Wash and drain wild rice. Place oil in large pot and sauté garlic and vegetables until translucent. Add lentils, wild rice, thyme, cumin, bay leaves, and broth. Bring to a boil, lower heat, cover, and simmer for approximately 1 hour or until wild rice is cooked and splits open.

Roasted Sweet Potatoes

This is a powerhouse of vitamin A.

2 large sweet potatoes (approximately 1 pound total weight)
1 tablespoon canola oil
6 slices turkey bacon
½ cup walnut pieces

Makes approximately 2½ cups.

Preheat oven to 350°F. Wash and dry sweet potatoes. Cut into 1-inch pieces. Place in bowl and toss with canola oil to coat. Cut turkey bacon into small pieces. Add turkey bacon and walnuts to potatoes, and toss to mix. Place on ungreased sheet pan and place in oven for approximately 45 minutes until potatoes are soft and bacon and walnuts are crispy.

Salmon Salad

This is high in protein, omega-3 fats, vitamin A, potassium, and fiber.

1 7½-ounce can pink salmon
1 6-ounce jar marinated artichoke hearts
1 cup chopped cooked broccoli
2 tablespoons lemon juice
2 tablespoons olive oil
½ teaspoon dried thyme
½ teaspoon dried oregano
½ teaspoon onion powder
2 tablespoons chopped capers

Makes 2¾ cups.

Drain salmon and flake with a fork. Drain and chop artichoke hearts. Combine flaked salmon, chopped artichokes, broccoli, lemon juice, olive oil, thyme, oregano, onion powder, and capers. Serve over mixed greens or in a whole wheat pita pocket or whole wheat wrap with lettuce and tomato.

Turkey and Spinach Meatballs

These are high in protein, vitamin A, and folacin, with some calcium, magnesium, and niacin.

> 1¼ pounds ground turkey
> 1 10-ounce package frozen chopped spinach, thawed and drained of
>   liquids
> 8 ounces fat-free ricotta
> 1 teaspoon salt
> 1 teaspoon hot sauce

Makes thirty 1-inch meatballs.

Preheat oven to 350°F. Combine ground turkey, spinach, ricotta, salt, and hot sauce. Roll into 1-inch meatballs, and place on sheet pan. Bake for approximately 15 minutes or until juices run clear. Make into smaller meatballs for hors d'oeuvres.

Fruit Soup

The key to a great fruit soup is using really ripe fruits. You can also substitute frozen fruits of your choice. This version is rich in vitamin A, vitamin C, and potassium.

1 pint strawberries
1 mango
1 large banana
½ cantaloupe
1 cup orange juice

Makes approximately 4¾ cups.

Wash strawberries and trim off stems. Peel mango and banana and cut into small pieces. Peel and seed cantaloupe. Cut into small pieces. Place all cut fruits and orange juice into blender or food processor and blend until smooth. Chill and serve.

10

Eating Well After Pregnancy

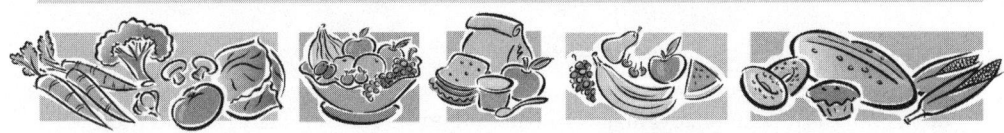

After your pregnancy, you are most likely going to devote most of your energy to caring for your new baby. If this is your first pregnancy, you will be adjusting to your new role as mother; if not, you will be juggling the needs of your other children with your new little one. Either way, the time after a baby is born is a time when women are often thinking about caring for others more than themselves. But caring for your own health now is also very important as your body recovers from pregnancy and as you begin breast-feeding, if you choose to do so. This chapter will discuss some of the primary nutritional concerns of new moms, such as these:

- Making the decision to breast- or bottle-feed
- Special nutritional needs while breast-feeding
- Losing the added weight of pregnancy
- Transitioning to a healthy diet after pregnancy

Your body has undergone some amazing changes and now has to readjust. But you've also made some changes in your behavior and become more conscious about what you eat. In this chapter I will give you a plan for turning the healthy habits you've worked so hard to cultivate during pregnancy into good nutrition for your future health.

Choosing to Breast-Feed or Bottle-Feed

One of the first and most important decisions that new mothers make is whether to breast-feed or bottle-feed their babies. In fact, you should make this decision *before* giving birth, because the first feeding should happen immediately after delivery. While the decision is a personal one that may include many factors, it is almost universally agreed by health authorities all over the world that breast-feeding is the healthiest choice for mothers and their babies. Here's why.

Advantages for Babies

Breast milk offers more advantages to babies than infant formula can. The widespread recognition that breast milk is best for babies is based on extensive research about the role of breast-feeding and health.

• *The best nutrients.* Breast milk is naturally suited for an infant's nutritional needs. It has the right mix of nutrients that babies need to grow and develop. It contains the right proportion of proteins, and its proteins are made of the right "building blocks"—amino acids—that are needed to construct the tissues of your baby's growing body. Breast milk also has the healthiest carbohydrates including some large, slowly digested carbohydrates that help to moderate blood sugar levels. These carbohydrates also serve as food for good bacteria, encouraging them to grow in a baby's digestive tract, which is a critical part of setting up a healthy digestive system. Breast milk also has a lot of good fats, such as omega-3 fatty acids, which may have benefits for a baby's brain development.

• *Tailor-made nutrition.* The contents of breast milk change as the baby gets older, and they even change from the beginning of a feeding to the end. Instead of a standardized formula, the baby receives nutrition suited to his special nutritional needs.

• *Immune protection.* Breast milk contains several factors that are thought to help a baby's naturally weak immune system. It contains proteins and antibodies that help to fight infections and promote immune system development. It even con-

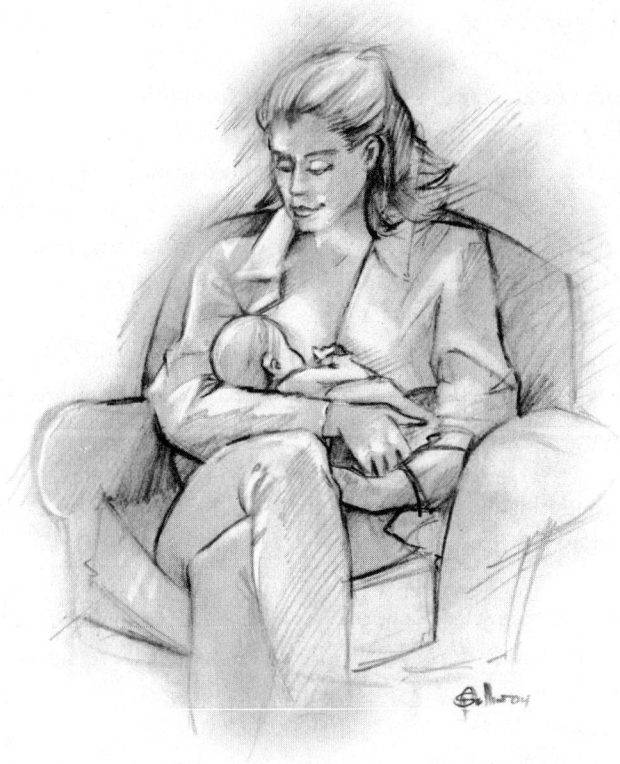

tains live cells and chemicals from a mother's immune system that can help protect her baby. Several studies have found that breast-feeding offers protection against certain infections as well as allergies.

• *Closeness with Mom.* Another, often overlooked, advantage of breast-feeding is the bond it produces between mother and child. Though it is difficult to study the effects that early experiences in infanthood have on child development, the close contact and interaction between mother and child that takes place during breast-feeding may help encourage emotional and cognitive development. Several different studies have found that breast-fed babies perform slightly better in cognitive tests even after infancy.

Advantages for Moms

Breast-feeding offers some important benefits for mothers, too.

• *Faster recovery.* Lactation—the production of milk—is the natural completion of the reproductive cycle after pregnancy and birth. The suckling of your baby shortly after delivery stimulates the release of oxytocin, a hormone that contracts the uterus and reduces bleeding, helping your body recover faster from delivery.

• *Easier weight loss.* During pregnancy, the body adds about six to eight pounds of body weight in anticipation of the energy requirements of breast-feeding. The production of milk in a lactating woman burns about 500 calories a day. Not all studies have shown that breast-feeding promotes weight loss—it also depends on a woman's food intake and physical activity level—but the added energy expenditure of nursing may help you lose your pregnancy weight.

• *Psychological benefits.* The hormones released during breast-feeding—oxytocin and prolactin—have been shown to stimulate maternal feelings and a sense of well-being.

• *Reduced disease risk.* Women who breast-feed have lower incidences of breast, uterine, and ovarian cancers. Lactation lowers estrogen levels in the body, and lifetime exposure to estrogen is a risk factor for these cancers. The longer you nurse, the greater the benefit. Breast-feeding also increases bone density, reducing the risk of osteoporosis and fractures later in life.

• *Less guesswork.* Women who breast-feed generally have an easier time knowing when their baby is full and has had enough. Studies have shown that bottle-fed infants consume more calories than they need, an early example of overeating that may be linked to overweight later in life. When you nurse, your breasts have a natural mechanism for stimulating and shutting off milk production. The contents of your breast milk even change as your feeding progresses, matching your baby's nutritional needs. With breast-feeding, you don't have to worry about choosing a formula and measuring the right amount. And it saves you the sizable expense and hassle of buying formulas, bottles, and nipples.

The federal government listed as one of its goals in its *Healthy People 2010* report to have 75 percent of women breast-feeding in the United States. Recent polls by the American Academy of Pediatrics (AAP) show that we are close to that goal: more than 71 percent of children have ever been breast-fed. However, our population is behind the goal on maintaining breast-feeding for the long term. The AAP recommends breast-feeding babies exclusively (without supplemental formula) for twelve months of life. Breast milk is enough to sustain them by itself until they are four to six months old, after which solid foods can be fed.

How Lactation Works

Your body's ability to produce and provide milk to your baby is controlled by hormones in your body, primarily one called prolactin. Levels of this hormone rise after delivery, enabling you to feed your baby immediately. Milk is produced automatically at first, but in order to continue producing milk you need the stimulation of your baby's sucking (or similar stimulation for a breast pump), which releases prolactin. Without stimulation at least once a day starting from a few days after delivery, women lose the ability to nurse. Another hormone, oxytocin, sets in motion the release of milk from ducts in your breast, sometimes called "letting down." Oxytocin is also stimulated by sucking, but even seeing your baby or hearing her cry can release the hormone and cause milk to flow.

In the first few days after delivery, your milk is yellowish and thick; this protein- and antibody-rich first milk is called colostrum. Because early milk is particularly high in nutrients for the newborn, I encourage women to try breast-feeding immediately after delivery and during the first days or weeks of their baby's life, even if they are not able to continue breast-feeding for the long term. The colostrum will turn into a light yellow or whitish milk after two to four days. Most women produce more than enough milk to feed a baby. The actual volume of milk you produce varies according to how much your baby demands—a very convenient system!

Tips for Breast-Feeding

Even though breast-feeding is a natural process for your body, it may not feel natural or come to you easily. Nursing may cause slight pain and discomfort at first, but once you get used to the sensation, breast-feeding shouldn't hurt as long as you position your baby correctly. Place him directly facing your chest and, when his mouth is open, pull him close to your breast. He should be able to latch on with his mouth, and his sucking should cause you to feel pressure and pulling. It's fine to shift positions for your own comfort—the important thing is to keep your baby directly facing you in any position you choose. Pain or cracked nipples are often a sign of incorrect positioning.

Most hospitals offer help for new mothers who are learning to breast-feed—take advantage of these services after your delivery. There are also certified lactation consultants who can help you breast-feed. Ask your doctor or find one through the International Lactation Consultant Association (ilca.org). You can also get help from books specifically about breast-feeding, such as *The Nursing Mother's Companion* by Kathleen Huggins.

New mothers often want some kind of a schedule or guideline about when to feed. But in reality, the best time to feed is when your baby is hungry. As a new mother, it's good to begin to pay attention to your baby's hunger cues. These include lip smacking, thrusting of the tongue, hands moving to the mouth, and rooting (the head turning with mouth open). Begin feeding as soon as you see these signs rather than waiting until your baby becomes distressed or cries, which may interfere with proper feeding. Most babies feed every two to three hours, but some young babies feed more often. They also may want to feed more frequently at some times and less frequently at others. By four days, babies should be feeding no fewer than eight to twelve times or more every twenty-four hours. You'll be able to see your baby swallowing, and your breasts should feel softer after the feeding. Try to feed ten to twenty minutes at each breast, so your baby can receive the hindmilk that appears several minutes into the feeding; it has a high fat content that helps growth and proper weight gain.

The Working Mom

Returning to work can be a major hurdle for a woman who wants to continue breast-feeding. Though your work schedule can get in the way of nursing, it is not necessarily a barrier. You can use a breast pump to produce milk throughout the day, which can be stored and bottle-fed to your baby while you're out. You can purchase an electric breast pump and a double-pumping kit that allow you to extract milk from both breasts at once. A breast pump will also help you maintain your milk supply for the times when you can feed your baby directly, because your breasts need to be stimulated to continue making milk.

Many workplaces have special rooms available to lactating mothers—if yours does not, try to find a private place. Don't be afraid to raise the issue with your employer to advocate for better facilities, because making demands will help other new mothers to have their needs met.

You can store the milk in a refrigerator or cooler for your baby to have the next day. Milk can be refrigerated for up to seventy-two hours, or it can be frozen and then thawed in warm water (not in the microwave, which can destroy nutrients in the milk). Refrigeration is better, as long as you don't need to store milk for long periods of time, because freezing can destroy immune cells and other components that help protect your baby from infections. Breast-feed your baby in the morning, after you return from work, during the evening, and on weekends as often as you can. If possible, visit your baby at home or at your day-care facility on your lunch break on workdays. But if you're away all day, plan on pumping milk two to three times a day—less for an older infant who is also eating solid foods.

During the first weeks and months after your pregnancy, you can take advantage of your maternity leave and the abundance of milk your body produces by storing extra milk for times when you won't be able to breast-feed (again, frozen milk is not ideal but can be a convenient way to stockpile milk for later use). Some women can pump one breast while their baby feeds at the other.

The Combination Approach

Health authorities such as the American Academy of Pediatrics advise women to breast-feed exclusively for the first year of life. But what if breast-feeding for a year seems impossible? Unfortunately, women may feel discouraged from breast-feeding at all if they can't live up to these standards. But breast-feeding is not "all or nothing"; if you can't breast-feed exclusively you should still breast-feed as much as you can. I recommend trying to breast-feed as much as possible in the first few weeks and months of your baby's life, without relying on a bottle (it's important for your baby to get used to the feeling of your breast instead of an artificial nipple). If you return to work or can no longer spend time feeding all day, try pumping and storing your milk. And if that can't cover your baby's needs, try to breast-feed in the morning and at night while supplementing with formula during the day. The bottom line is that every time you breast-feed is a positive step for your baby's health.

Nutrition During Lactation

When you are nursing, your body is like a manufacturing plant making all the food your baby needs to grow and thrive for the first four to six months of life. This is no mean feat. It takes energy to make all that food, even more energy than was needed during pregnancy. If this is surprising to you, consider this: your baby will

The Best Way to Bottle-Feed

If you bottle-feed your baby, you can be assured that reputable commercial formulas follow standardized guidelines for quality and nutrition. Although formula can't match all the components of breast milk, formula manufacturers are constantly striving to make it closer nutritionally to nature. Most formulas are based on cow's milk and then altered so that they are closer to human milk (babies should *never* be given cow's milk instead of formula). For instance, the butterfat from milk is taken out and replaced with a mix of vegetable oils and animal fats that better match the fats found in human milk. The American Academy of Pediatrics recommends using iron-fortified formulas to prevent iron deficiencies. Formula companies have recently been adding DHA, a type of omega-3 fatty acid, to formulas, which some evidence shows may have a positive effect on brain development.

Special protein hydrolysate formulas are available for infants who have difficulty digesting milk protein. Some formulas are also based on soy—these are sometimes recommended for infants who lack the enzyme that digests lactose, or milk sugar. But soy contains isoflavones, chemicals in plants that can mimic the activity of the hormone estrogen, and there has been some concern that these hormonelike substances can alter the normal development of an infant. A formula based on cow's milk is the best choice for most infants.

If you bottle-feed exclusively, you can take special care to foster the close mother-to-child contact that breast-feeding provides. You can make the experience of bottle-feeding more interactive by holding your baby as close as possible, allowing her to feel the warmth of your skin as she feeds, talking to her, and trying to hold eye contact so she can see your facial expressions.

Studies have shown that formula-fed infants consume more calories than they need—perhaps because parents feel their babies must finish a bottle—and lack the natural portion regulation of breast-feeding. Learn to follow your baby's cues that show she is hungry or satisfied. Formulas offer guidelines for how much babies should be fed every day, but it's better to let your baby decide when she's had enough.

grow as much in the first four to six months of life as he grew the entire nine months of your pregnancy. Babies don't need to even begin eating other foods until they are four to six months old, so their mother's milk provides all the energy they need to double their birth weight!

Breast-feeding is designed to provide nutrition to your baby without you having to put much thought into it. Even mothers who are nutritionally deprived can nurse their babies, but mothers who have better diets can provide better-quality milk to their babies. Your body can't make milk from nothing—it requires the raw materials necessary to manufacture food that's fit for your baby. Breast milk is made from water, fats, protein, and carbohydrates, as well as some vitamins and minerals. Your goal as you nurse is to eat a nutrient-rich, balanced diet to make all these ingredients available for milk.

Some components of breast milk can vary according to what you eat, so it's better for your baby if you eat nutrient-rich foods. Fats are one example. When a mother eats a diet high in unsaturated fats, there will be more unsaturated fat in her milk; when she eats a diet high in unhealthy trans fats, these also show up in greater quantities. To maximize the good fats available to your baby, continue to choose unsaturated fats, and limit sources of saturated and trans fats. Levels of some vitamins and minerals are also affected by the mother's diet. Some nutrients may be pulled from your own body's stores for your milk, so staying nourished is important for your own health, too.

- *Calories.* You should plan on eating about 500 extra calories beyond what you were used to eating before pregnancy—about the amount in a sandwich. But what about the extra fat I told you was being stored in your body in preparation for nursing? The recommendation to eat 500 more calories assumes you will also be using about 170 calories a day from the fat reserves stored from pregnancy. If you are worried about losing weight after your pregnancy, keep in mind that any weight loss should be gradual so as not to interfere with milk production; you won't have to restrict calories severely because nursing will burn many of them for you. Your need for extra calories will gradually taper after about six months of nursing when your baby begins to eat solid foods and your milk production lessens slightly.

- *Protein.* Lactating women should continue eating extra protein as they did when they were pregnant—a total of 70 grams per day.

- *Vitamins and minerals.* The dietary reference intakes (DRIs) set by the Institute of Medicine are even higher for certain vitamins and minerals during nursing than during pregnancy. Much of the additional levels of these nutrients will be covered by the extra food you eat while you are nursing—provided those extra calories come from nutrient-rich foods. As you can see from the Table 10.1, eating a variety of lean meats, whole grains, legumes, nuts, seeds, fruits, vegetables, and seafood should cover all your bases.

• *Healthy fats*. Babies require essential fats to develop properly. There are two kinds of essential fats: omega-6 and omega-3. Many health experts believe that the current American diet has an unhealthy imbalance of these two forms of fat, favoring omega-6 fats and lacking in omega-3 fats. Omega-3 fatty acids, especially a form called DHA, aid in the development of the nervous system, reduce inflammation, and may even help babies sleep and prevent allergies.

One ongoing study on the effects of supplementing breast-feeding moms with omega-3 fatty acids found that their children did slightly better on tests of mental acuity when they were four years old than children of women supplemented with omega-6 fats. The exact relationship between these fats and intelligence is complicated and requires further study to make any conclusions. However, because DHA is a natural component of a healthy diet and a necessity for proper development, it's wise for women to include extra DHA in their diets while they are nursing. Fish is one of the best sources of omega-3 fatty acids, but women who are breast-feeding should continue to follow the same precautions about fish intake as they did while pregnant to avoid high mercury levels (see Chapter 5). You can continue taking a daily DHA/fish oil supplement and supplement your fish intake with DHA-enriched eggs. Flaxseed, soy, walnuts, and canola oil also contain a form of fat that can be turned into omega-3 fats in the body, though how well these foods substitute for more direct forms of omega-3s is not clear.

• *Water*. Nursing mothers need to replenish the fluids they lose from milk production. Try to drink extra water throughout the day. Eating lots of fruits and vegetables, which are made mostly of water, also helps boost hydration. Staying hydrated may also help with constipation, a common complaint of women after childbirth.

• *Vegetarian diets*. Women who are vegan or vegetarian should consult their doctors or see a nutritionist to make sure they are getting the balanced nutrition they need to breast-feed. Vegetarians are particularly vulnerable to vitamin B_{12} deficiency, because this vitamin is not found in plant sources of protein. In 2001, the

Table 10.1 Dietary Reference Intakes (DRIs) During Lactation

NUTRIENT	DRI FOR PREGNANCY	DRI FOR LACTATION	SELECTED FOOD SOURCES
Biotin	30 mcg/day	35 mcg/day	Concentrated in liver; small amounts in vegetables and meats
Choline	450 mg/day	550 mg/day	Milk, liver, eggs, peanuts
Vitamin C	85 mg/day	120 mg/day	Citrus fruits, tomatoes, potatoes, brussels sprouts, broccoli, cauliflower, cabbage, spinach
Vitamin A	770 mcg/day	1,300 mcg (2,565 IU)/day	Liver, dairy products, fish, dark fruits, leafy vegetables
Vitamin B_6	1.5 mg/day	1.6 mg/day	Fortified cereals, organ meats, fortified soy-based meat substitutes
Vitamin B_{12}	2.6 mcg/day	2.8 mcg/day	Fortified cereals, meat, fish, poultry
Riboflavin (B_2)	1.4 mg/day	1.6 mg/day	Milk, bread products, fortified cereals
Pantothenic acid	6 mg/day	7 mg/day	Potatoes, oats, cereals, tomato products, liver, kidney, yeast, eggs, broccoli, whole grains
Vitamin E	15 mg/day	19 mg/day	Vegetable oils, unprocessed grains, nuts, seeds, fruits, meats
Chromium	30 mcg/day	45 mcg/day	Some cereals, poultry, meat, fish
Copper	1,000 mcg/day	1,300 mcg/day	Seafood, nuts, seeds, wheat bran, whole grains, cocoa
Iodine	220 mcg/day	290 mcg/day	Foods from the sea, iodized salt
Manganese	2 mg/day	2.6 mg/day	Nuts, legumes, tea, whole grains
Selenium	60 mcg/day	70 mcg/day	Found in a wide variety of plant foods; also organ meats, seafood
Zinc	11 mg/day	12 mg/day	Fortified cereals, meats, some seafood

Centers for Disease Control and Prevention issued a warning regarding two cases of vitamin B_{12} deficiency in infants who were breast-fed by vegetarian mothers. These babies had serious developmental delays, which could be only partially corrected by later supplementation with vitamin B_{12}. Any nursing mom who is vegetarian or vegan should take a B_{12} supplement and should review her diet with her doctor to see if she needs to make additional adjustments. Women who consume no or few dairy products may also need a vitamin D supplement.

Things to Avoid While Breast-Feeding

During the period when you are breast-feeding, your baby is exposed to any potentially harmful agents that find their way into your milk. Some causes for concern include these:

- **Alcohol.** Alcohol shows up in breast milk. Breast-feeding moms should avoid alcohol except for a small occasional drink, and they should avoid nursing for two hours after the drink.

- **Caffeine.** Caffeine also travels into breast milk and has been known to cause signs of agitation and sleeplessness in babies, so it's best to limit caffeine to the equivalent of one or two small cups of coffee a day, as you did when pregnant.

- **Smoking.** If you were a smoker and quit for your pregnancy, it's in your and your baby's best interest to avoid starting again. Nicotine and other chemicals make their way into breast milk, secondhand smoke is a known carcinogen for babies, and smoking is dangerous for your health. Smoking increases your risk of dying of cancer, heart disease, and lung disease, and a study conducted by the Centers for Disease Control found that smoking reduces women's lives by nearly fifteen years.

- **Medications.** Most medications are fine to take when breast-feeding, but there are some that may have an effect on a baby, especially certain treatments for mental disorders. It's important to talk to your doctor about any medications you take, as there may be safer alternatives that allow you to continue breast-feeding.

- **Fish and mercury.** Lactating women should continue following guidelines for avoiding high mercury levels in fish, listed in Chapter 5.

Can a Nursing Mother's Diet Cause Allergies or Intestinal Problems in Her Baby?

There is much controversy as to whether the foods a woman eats while nursing can cause allergies, asthma, or intestinal discomfort in her baby. The idea that foods you eat may cause sensitivities or fussiness in your baby is strong in popular culture, but in reality fussiness is a normal part of being a baby, and the foods you eat have much less effect than you may think. Evidence does suggest that some cases of colic—persistent long-term crying spells and irritability—may be eased by cutting cow's milk out of the mother's diet. Gas is absolutely normal for babies, but if yours has excessive gas and discomfort, you can try cutting back on foods that typically cause gas and bloating in you.

Breast-feeding has been linked with lower rates of allergic diseases in infants, including food allergies. But for babies who have a family history of food allergies or allergic disease, it's often recommended that breast-feeding mothers cut back on common allergens such as cow's milk, eggs, or peanuts, which can find their way into breast milk. However, a review of several studies that examined allergen-restricted diets during nursing found that eczema was the only condition that showed any noticeable reduction from a restricted diet.

A small percentage of babies experience a marked change in behavior or a health problem after their mothers eat certain foods. If you notice symptoms such as rash, wheezing, severe irritability, intestinal upset, diarrhea, constipation, vomiting, or other acute health problems after a feeding, it may be a sign of food allergy. Cut the suspected food from your diet for a couple of weeks to see if the symptoms go away. Make sure you are making up for any nutrients you lose from the restricted foods, because your nutrition can potentially be compromised by removing important protein sources from your diet.

Losing Weight After Pregnancy

Most women gradually shed the extra weight they gained during pregnancy. As I mentioned in Chapter 7, the majority of the weight you gained was not simply stored fat. Some of it was from your baby and some from the placenta. Nearly one-third of it came from extra fluids your body produced, and this weight will gradually diminish once your body returns to normal and those fluids and extra tissues are not needed. But losing the fat you did gain can be tricky, especially for those who tend to put on extra fat during pregnancy or retain it afterward.

How fast should you lose weight? Our magazines are filled with photos of celebrity women who, just a few weeks after having a baby, appear on a red carpet to show off their figures, which seem to have miraculously returned to prepregnancy thinness. These women offer a sometimes unreachable—and unhealthy—goal to the average woman just recovering from a pregnancy. Because these women rely on their bodies for work, they are under tremendous pressure to lose weight even if it is at an unsafe pace. And these women have the financial resources to make it happen, with nannies, personal trainers, and chefs at the ready. The reality is that it will take time to lose weight, and depending on how much you gained, you should think of your weight loss stretching over six months or more. Losing about one pound per week, or four pounds a month, is a healthy pace.

Many women are motivated to lose any extra fat for looks, but there are important health reasons why it's good to shed any extra pounds you gained during pregnancy (unless you were underweight to begin with). Here is a common scenario: a woman gains a little weight during her first pregnancy and finds it difficult to lose the weight in the next months. She gets pregnant again before she is able to get back to her normal weight. She gains the same amount of weight or more in her second pregnancy, this time finishing at an even higher weight than before. The additive effect of weight gain over multiple pregnancies can nudge her into the "overweight" or "obese" category by the time she finishes having children, putting her long-term health at risk.

Studies examining weight loss and weight retention after pregnancy have found that women who control the number of calories they eat and who exercise regularly have an easier time losing weight. Rather than looking for a particular weight-loss "program" over the next few months, focus on setting up healthy habits that you plan to keep for life. Everybody's metabolism slows down with age, and a slower-running engine needs increasingly less fuel. Making small, gradual adjustments in how many calories you eat and how much physical activity you engage in will be a lifelong process. Choose activities you want to pursue for the long term, and choose eating habits you can maintain, rather than temporary fad diets. I would recommend specialized diet programs by a registered dietitian or a program such as Weight Watchers for women who need individual help and structure to get rid of excess weight—and only if the program has a plan for integrating changes into your life over the long term.

If you are planning to have another child, ideally you should wait until you have lost most or all of your pregnancy weight before conceiving. Pregnancy puts your body under stress, and your next pregnancy will be healthier if you give your metabolism a chance to return to normal.

Exercising After Pregnancy

Your body needs to recover from the stress of pregnancy and delivery, and it's common for physicians to recommend that women refrain from any serious exercise until their six-week postpartum checkup. But it's safe to gradually start returning to your prepregnancy activities or, if you were fairly sedentary before pregnancy, continue or increase the activity level you established while you were pregnant. Exercising regularly can help you set aside some personal time to care for yourself in the midst of the busyness of being a parent. It has also been shown to lower the risk of postpartum depression, as long as the activity you choose is not one that causes you emotional stress. And regular physical activity will help you avoid retaining your pregnancy weight. Talk to your doctor about the pace and intensity of activity you can expect to accomplish in the first few weeks—women with pregnancy complications may require more rest.

Walking with your baby in a stroller is a great way to continue staying physically active. More and more fitness and health-care centers are offering specialized postnatal exercise programs—and some of them even include baby, such as fitness walks with strollers, parent-baby aerobics, and even baby yoga. Check to see what's available in your area.

After childbirth, your abdominal muscles are loose from being stretched for so long, and they must be returned to their former length. You can help this process along by continuing to perform abdominal-tightening exercises such as the ones described and illustrated in Chapter 8. At first, this may involve simply lying on your back with knees bent with feet on the floor and pulling the muscles down toward your spine. Eventually you can start doing pelvic tilts and after the third day, curl-ups. (First make sure that the center seam between your abdominal muscles has returned to a two-finger width.) Start doing each exercise only a few times, and work up to more repetitions.

Use your lower abdominal muscles to stabilize your pelvis during progressively difficult leg movements. Lie on your back with knees bent and feet on the floor.

Begin by sliding your heels out but stop if your pelvis moves up before your knees are straight. When you can maintain a neutral pelvic tilt while fully extending your legs, progress to bicycling with both legs, bringing them over your waist one at a time. Then, legs lifted and knees slightly bent, lower both legs slowly while maintaining correct alignment of pelvis and spine. For a final challenge, bring the legs up straight and lower slowly to a forty-five-degree angle, using the abdominals to keep the lower back from arching.

It's good to consult with a personal trainer at a gym to make sure you are doing any exercises correctly. Classes designed for building abdominal strength, such as Pilates mat classes, can be helpful but may be too strenuous in the first weeks after delivery.

You also want to continue performing pelvic floor contractions immediately after delivery, to help these muscles regain their shape and tightness. Without strengthening the pelvic floor, you could be more prone to urinary incontinence, and your muscles may have difficulty withstanding pressures from weight-bearing exercises.

Recovering After Cesarean Section

Women who have cesarean sections will need to take more rest and expect a longer recovery period—after all, you've just had major surgery as well as given birth to a baby. The typical recovery period for this surgery is six weeks, but follow your doctor's advice about what you can do when. During your recovery, you should refrain from lifting anything heavier than your baby, avoid climbing stairs many times in a day, take frequent naps, and avoid much activity beyond brief periods of walking. Practicing deep breathing and slow, gentle movements can help stimulate the muscles and internal organs of your body as you recover.

You can start doing passive abdominal exercises immediately to help regain strength—as you are lying down, simply pull the muscles down and in toward the spine. You can transition to a modified curl-up by propping your back up with pillows. With your knees bent, tuck your chin down and tilt your pelvis back toward your upper body, flattening the curve of your back. Reach your arms forward, and bring them forward to your knees as you contract your abdominals. Then relax back to the pillows. From the same propped-up position, you can stimulate your leg muscles by alternately bending and straightening each leg. Once you are feeling better, you can graduate to full curl-ups and other abdominal exercises.

Good Nutrition for the Long Term

You put a lot of effort into taking care of your body and your health during your pregnancy. You may have made these changes to benefit your baby, but they benefited you, too. Now that your pregnancy is over, you can take the opportunity to keep following some of those good habits to help you stay healthy and avoid diseases that are caused by an unhealthy lifestyle.

- *Balance.* Continue to eat a balanced diet containing a variety of the healthiest foods from each food group. Your need for protein and dairy products is not so high after pregnancy and lactation, but in general you want to continue choosing foods that provide a mix of carbohydrates, healthy fats, and protein and an array of vitamins and minerals.

- *Better carbohydrates.* Keep eating whole grains and other healthy sources of carbohydrates. Maintaining healthy blood sugar levels can keep your metabolism running smoothly and prevent high blood sugar and diabetes. Learn to look for added sugars in the foods you eat and avoid or limit them as much as possible.

- *More fruits and vegetables.* Add fruits and vegetables to your diet whenever you can—aim for five or more servings per day. These foods provide fiber, water, vitamins, minerals, and hundreds of other compounds called phytochemicals that may have important benefits for health, including cancer prevention.

- *The best fats.* Avoid unhealthy saturated and trans fats, and eat foods rich in healthy unsaturated fats such as plant oils and nuts. Once lactation is over, you can safely add more fish, which contains omega-3 fats that may help reduce your risk of heart disease, may ease arthritis and other inflammatory conditions, and may even help prevent depression. Choose protein sources that are low in saturated fats, such as nuts, seeds, legumes, low-fat and fat-free dairy products, fish, and lean meats.

- *Supplements for insurance.* Continue to take a daily folic acid supplement if you may have another child. Rather than a prenatal vitamin, you may want to take a regular adult multivitamin as "insurance" to prevent deficiencies. Choose a standard formula without a lot of untested herbal ingredients, and never take high doses.

• *Convenient nutrition.* Always keep nutritious snacks within reach. As parenting takes up more of your concentration, you will be tempted to reach for unhealthy foods that are convenient. Plan ahead and prepackage foods to take with you.

• *Calorie maintenance.* After pregnancy and lactation, your calorie needs change. Rather than trying to cut out one of the snacks or meals you were used to eating, try reducing portion sizes slightly all around. If you were drinking caloric beverages, try switching to plain water or other calorie-free drinks. Maintaining a healthy weight is a key part of long-term prevention of disease. And in today's environment of easily available, high-calorie foods, weight maintenance is an ongoing, lifelong reality. Get in the habit of paying attention to portion sizes, stop eating when you are nearly full, and don't finish large portions served at restaurants. Eat smaller portions of calorie-dense foods, such as sweets and baked goods, and larger portions of lower-calorie foods such as fruits and vegetables.

• *Physical activity.* Regular physical activity can help you maintain your weight and reduce your risk of cardiovascular disease and diabetes. Try some of the "active lifestyle" tips from Chapter 8, which can be incorporated into your daily routine without need for special exercise classes or equipment. You can now also take regular walks with your baby.

• *Good information.* Always seek out information about the foods you eat by reading food labels and asking for nutrition information at restaurants. It's also important to seek the best science-based advice about nutrition, rather than relying on fad diets or anecdote. I recommend reading a book such as *Eat, Drink, and Be Healthy* by my colleague Walter C. Willett, who draws on his extensive research to present guidelines for good health. While federal guidelines for diet are often plagued by politics, the 2005 *Dietary Guidelines for Americans* are much more closely matched with the research findings and recommendations of nutrition experts and offer special recommendations for different populations. They are summarized at health.gov/dietaryguidelines/dga2005/document/html/executive summary.htm. I also recommend consulting a dietitian for individualized nutrition expertise.

Finally, although I've been focusing on your health, taking these steps will benefit your baby, too. You are now your child's role model, and all of the things you do for your own health—choosing the healthiest foods, following a balanced diet, controlling the amount of food you eat, and engaging in regular physical activities—help to teach your child good habits by example. To learn more about how to feed your child during infancy, toddlerhood, and early childhood, see my book *Eat, Play, and Be Healthy: The Harvard Medical School Guide to Healthy Eating for Kids*. I hope you enjoy your new role as a mother and continue the efforts you made in pregnancy to care for your health and give your child the best start possible.

Nutrition After Pregnancy: The Bottom Line

After pregnancy, you may be overwhelmed by the joys and duties of parenthood, but it's important to take the good health habits you learned and keep practicing them for the long term. Remember the following:

- Choosing to breast-feed or bottle-feed is a personal decision with many possible factors, but health authorities agree that breast-feeding is best for a baby's health.
- During lactation, women have a higher need for calories, protein, and certain vitamins and minerals. You should stay well nourished while nursing and follow the same precautions and health habits that you did during pregnancy.
- Plan to lose your pregnancy weight over the course of several months, about four pounds per month. Don't severely cut back on calories (especially if you are breast-feeding), but instead monitor your weight loss and make small adjustments in your calorie intake or activity level if you are not losing weight.
- Gradually begin exercising after pregnancy, taking care to rebuild strength and tone in your abdominal and pelvic muscles.
- Continue to follow good eating habits to decrease your risk of developing heart disease, obesity, diabetes, and other lifestyle diseases while being the best role model you can be for your child.

References

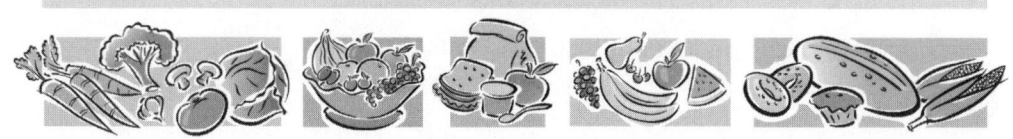

Introduction

American Dietetic Association. eatright.org.

Anderson, A. S. "Pregnancy as a Time for Dietary Change?" *Proceedings of the Nutrition Society* 60 (2001): 497–504.

Dietary Guidelines for Americans 2005. healthierus.gov/dietaryguidelines.

Harvard School of Public Health, Nutrition Source. hsph.harvard.edu/nutritionsource.

Walker, W. A., and Courtney Humphries. *Eat, Play, and Be Healthy: The Harvard Medical School Guide to Healthy Eating for Kids.* Chicago: McGraw-Hill, 2005.

Willett, W. C., and P. J. Skerrett. *Eat, Drink, and Be Healthy: The Harvard Medical School Guide to Healthy Eating.* New York: Simon and Schuster Source, 2001.

Chapter 1

March of Dimes. marchofdimes.org.

National Council on Alcoholism and Drug Dependence. ncadd.org.

National Drug and Alcohol Treatment Referral Service. niaaa.nih.gov/other/referral.

National Women's Health Information Center. "Fertility Awareness and Infertility." 4woman.gov/Pregnancy/infertility.cfm.

Norman, R. J., et al. "Improving Reproductive Performance in Overweight/Obese Women with Effective Weight Management." *Human Reproduction Update* 10, no. 3 (2004): 267–80.

Shrander-Stumpel, C. "Preconception Care: Challenge of the New Millennium?" *American Journal of Medical Genetics* 89 (1999): 58–61.

Substance Abuse Treatment Facility Locator. http://dasis3.samhsa.gov.

Watkins, M. L., et al. "Maternal Obesity and Risk for Birth Defects." *Pediatrics* 111 (2003): 1152–58.

Chapter 2

Bainbridge, David. *Making Babies: The Science of Pregnancy.* Cambridge, MA: Harvard University Press, 2001.

Blackburn, Susan, ed. *Maternal, Fetal, and Neonatal Physiology.* 2nd ed. St. Louis: Saunders, 2003.

Chapter 3

Bernstein, H., and D. Novak. "Fetal Nutrition and Imprinting." In *Nutrition in Pediatrics: Basic Science and Clinical Applications.* 3rd ed., edited by W. Allan Walker, John Watkins, and Christopher Duggan. Hamilton, ON: B. C. Decker, Inc., 2001.

Gillman, M. W. "Epidemiological Challenges in Studying the Fetal Origins of Adult Chronic Disease." *International Journal of Epidemiology* 31 (2002): 294–99.

Gluckman, P. D., and M. A. Hanson. "Developmental Origins of Disease Paradigm: A Mechanistic and Evolutionary Perspective." *Pediatric Research* 56, no. 3 (2004): 311–17.

Gluckman, Peter, and Mark Hanson. *The Fetal Matrix: Evolution, Development and Disease.* Cambridge, MA: Cambridge University Press, 2005.

Waterland, R. A., and C. Garza. "Potential Mechanisms of Metabolic Imprinting That Lead to Chronic Disease." *American Journal of Clinical Nutrition* 69 (1999): 179–97.

Chapter 4

American Dietetic Association. "Position of the American Dietetic Association: Nutrition and Lifestyle for a Healthy Pregnancy Outcome." *Journal of the American Dietetic Association* 102, no. 10 (October 2002): 1479–90.

American Dietetic Association. eatright.org.

Erick, Miriam. *Managing Morning Sickness: A Survival Guide for Pregnant Women.* Boulder, CO: Bull Publishing Co., 2004.

Hornstra, Gerard. "Essential Fatty Acids in Mothers and Their Neonates." *American Journal of Clinical Nutrition* Suppl. 71 (2000): 1262S–69S.

Kleinman, Ronald, ed. "Nutrition During Pregnancy." In *Pediatric Nutrition Handbook.* 5th ed. Elk Grove Village, IL: American Academy of Pediatrics, 2004.

Nutrition.gov, the U.S. Department of Agriculture website. nutrition.gov.

Scholl, Theresa O. "Maternal Nutrition and Pregnancy Outcome." In *Nutrition in Pediatrics: Basic Science and Clinical Applications.* 3rd ed., edited by W. Allan Walker, John Watkins, and Christopher Duggan. Hamilton, ON: B. C. Decker, Inc., 2001.

Scholl, Teresa O., and W. G. Johnson. "Folic Acid: Influence on the Outcome of Pregnancy." *American Journal of Clinical Nutrition* Suppl. 71 (2000): 1295S–303S.

Chapter 5

Buehle, B. A. "Interactions of Herbal Products with Conventional Medicines and Potential Impact on Pregnancy." *Birth Defects Research* 68 (2003): 494–95.

Center for Evaluation of Risks to Human Reproduction (CERHR). "Common Concerns and Exposures." http://cerhr.niehs.nih.gov/genpub/topics/ccae _index.html.

Center for Science in the Public Interest. Nutrition Action Newsletter. "Caffeine Corner." cspinet.org/nah/caffeine/caffeine_corner.htm.

Kharrazi, M., et al. "Environmental Tobacco Smoke and Pregnancy Outcome." *Epidemiology* 15, no. 6 (November 2004): 660–70.

Motherisk Program at the Hospital for Sick Children in Toronto. motherisk.org.

National Council on Alcoholism and Drug Dependence. ncadd.org.

National Drug and Alcohol Treatment Referral Service. niaaa.nih.gov/other/referral.

Substance Abuse Treatment Facility Locator. http://dasis3.samhsa.gov.

Syme, M. R., et al. "Drug Transfer and Metabolism by the Human Placenta." *Clinical Pharmacokinetics* 43, no. 8 (2004): 487–514.

U.S. Food and Drug Administration. "Mercury Levels in Commercial Fish and Shellfish." cfsan.fda.gov/%7Efrf/sea-mehg.html (accessed March 17, 2005).

U.S. Food and Drug Administration/Environmental Protection Agency. "What You Need to Know About Mercury in Fish and Shellfish, March 2004." cfsan.fda.gov/~dms/admehg3.html (accessed March 17, 2005).

Chapter 6

Centers for Disease Control and Prevention. "Recommendations to Prevent and Control Iron Deficiency in the United States." *Morbidity and Mortality Weekly Report* 47, RR-3 (April 3, 1998): 1–36.

Committee on Nutritional Status During Pregnancy and Lactation, Institute of Medicine. *Nutrition During Pregnancy: Part II: Nutrient Supplements.* Washington, DC: National Academics Press, 1990.

"Facts About Vitamin A and Retinoids." http://ods.od.nih.gov/factsheets/cc/vita.html (accessed February 7, 2005).

National Institutes of Health Office of Dietary Supplements. "Vitamin and Mineral Supplement Fact Sheets." http://ods.od.nih.gov/Health_Information/Vitamin_and_Mineral_Supplement_Fact_Sheets.aspx.

Picciano, M. F. "Pregnancy and Lactation: Physiological Adjustments, Nutritional Requirements and the Role of Dietary Supplements." *Journal of Nutrition* 133, no. 6 (June 2003): 1997S–2002S.

U.S. Food and Drug Administration/Center for Food Safety and Applied Nutrition. "Dietary Supplements." cfsan.fda.gov/~dms/supplmnt.html.

Wainwright, P. E. "Dietary Essential Fatty Acids and Brain Function: A Developmental Perspective on Mechanisms." *Proceedings of the National Academy of Sciences* 61, no. 1 (2002): 61–69.

Chapter 7

Abrams, B., S. L. Altman, and K. E. Pickett. "Pregnancy Weight Gain: Still Controversial." *American Journal of Clinical Nutrition* Suppl. 71, no. 5 (May 2000): 1233S–41S.

Committee on Nutritional Status During Pregnancy and Lactation, Institute of Medicine. *Nutrition During Pregnancy: Part I: Weight Gain.* Washington, DC: National Academics Press, 1990.

Galtier-Dereure, F., C. Boegner, and J. Bringer. "Obesity and Pregnancy: Complications and Cost." *American Journal of Clinical Nutrition* Suppl. 71, no. 5 (May 2000): 1242S–48S.

Hamaoui, Elie, and Michael Hamaoui. "Nutritional Assessment and Support During Pregnancy." *Gastroenterology Clinics of North America* 32 (2003): 59–121.

Weight-Control Information Network, an information service of the National Institute of Diabetes and Digestive and Kidney Diseases (NIDDK). http://win.niddk.nih.gov/index.htm.

Chapter 8

American College of Obstetricians and Gynecologists. "ACOG Committee Opinion No. 267: Exercise During Pregnancy and the Postpartum Period." *Obstetrics and Gynecology* 99 (2002): 171–73.

Clap, J. F., III. "The Effects of Maternal Exercise on Fetal Oxygenation and Feto-Placental Growth." *European Journal of Obstetrics & Gynecology and Reproductive Biology* 110 (2003): S80–S85.

Gunderson, E. P. "Nutrition During Pregnancy for the Physically Active Woman." *Clinical Obstetrics and Gynecology* 46, no. 2 (2003): 390–402.

Noble, Elizabeth. *Essential Exercises for the Childbearing Year.* 3rd ed. Boston: Houghton Mifflin Company, 1988.

Wang, T. W., and B. S. Apgar. "Exercise During Pregnancy." *American Family Physician* 7, no. 8 (1998): 1846–52.

Chapter 10

American Academy of Pediatrics Committee on Drugs. "The Transfer of Drugs and Other Chemicals into Human Milk." *Pediatrics* 108, no. 3 (September 2001): 776–89.

Anderson, J. W. et al. "Breast-Feeding and Cognitive Development." *American Journal of Clinical Nutrition* 70 (1999): 525–35.

4woman.gov, the National Women's Health Information Center. "Breastfeeding—Best for Baby, Best for Mom." 4woman.gov/breastfeeding.

Healthy People 2010 home page. healthypeople.gov.

Huggins, Kathleen. *The Nursing Mothers Companion.* 5th ed., Boston: Harvard Common Press, 2005.

International Lactation Consultant Association. ilca.org.

Kleinman, Ronald. "Breastfeeding." In *Pediatric Nutrition Handbook.* 5th ed. Elk Grove Village, IL: American Academy of Pediatrics, 2004.

Kramer M. S., and R. Kakuma. "Maternal Dietary Antigen Avoidance During Pregnancy and/or Lactation for Preventing or Treating Atopic Disease in the Child." *The Cochrane Database of Systematic Reviews* no. 4 (2003).

La Leche League International. lalecheleague.org.

Lawrence, R., and R. M. Lawrence. "Approach to Breastfeeding." In *Nutrition in Pediatrics: Basic Science and Clinical Applications.* 3rd ed., edited by W. Allan Walker, John Watkins, and Christopher Duggan. Hamilton, ON: B. C. Decker, Inc., 2001.

Lightdale, R. J., et al. "Human Milk: Nutritional Properties." In *Nutrition in Pediatrics: Basic Science and Clinical Applications.* 3rd ed., edited by W. Allan Walker, John Watkins, and Christopher Duggan. Hamilton, ON: B. C. Decker, Inc., 2001.

Picciano, M. F. "Pregnancy and Lactation: Physiological Adjustments, Nutritional Requirements and the Role of Dietary Supplements." *Journal of Nutrition* 133, no. 6 (June 2003): 1997S–2002S.

Walker, W. A., and Courtney Humphries. *Eat, Play, and Be Healthy: The Harvard Medical School Guide to Healthy Eating for Kids.* Chicago: McGraw-Hill, 2005.

Willett, W. C., and P. J. Skerrett. *Eat, Drink, and Be Healthy: The Harvard Medical School Guide to Healthy Eating.* New York: Simon and Schuster Source, 2001.

Ziegler, E. E., et al. "The Term Infant." In *Nutrition in Pediatrics: Basic Science and Clinical Applications.* 3rd ed., edited by W. Allan Walker, John Watkins, and Christopher Duggan. Hamilton, ON: B. C. Decker, Inc., 2001.

Index

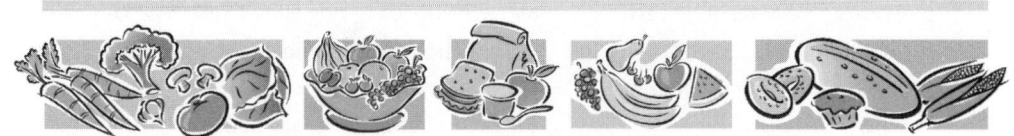

Page numbers in **bold** refer to recipes.

DA MAY 1 9 2006